A Conversation about Healthy Eating

A Conversation about Healthy Eating

Nicholas A. Lesica

ᴬUCLPRESS

First published in 2017 by
UCL Press
University College London
Gower Street
London WC1E 6BT

Available to download free: www.ucl.ac.uk/ucl-press

A CIP catalogue record for this book is available
from The British Library.

ISBN: 978–1–911576–77–8 (Hbk.)
ISBN: 978–1–911576–76–1 (Pbk.)
ISBN: 978–1–911576–75–4 (PDF)
ISBN: 978–1–911576–78–5 (epub)
ISBN: 978–1–911576–79–2 (mobi)
ISBN: 978–1–911576–80–8 (html)
DOI: https://doi.org/10.14324/111.9781911576754

Acknowledgements

I would like to thank the following people for their help during the writing and publishing process:

My wife Tara, for insisting that I do something useful for once and supporting me throughout;

The organizers of the 2016 Accountability Strategy Summit, especially Marta, for helpful discussions;

My friends at the Dulwich Squash Club, especially Andy, Mikey P., Davey, Mikey A., Josh, Mark, Tomas, Giles and Pete, for their suggestions and encouragement;

The spa team at the St. Pancras Renaissance Hotel, for providing an oasis of calm in which much of the reading and thinking for this book was done;

Chris and the rest of the team at UCL Press, for being open minded about the non-traditional format.

Contents

Introduction I

OK, this is really more of a glorified preface but I wanted to be sure that you didn't skip it. I tend to skip prefaces because I prefer my experience of a book to be unbiased. I don't want to know anyone else's thoughts about a book – not even the author's – until I've finished reading it and formed thoughts of my own. But this approach does have its risks: sometimes my expectations are wrong and I end up disappointed by a book that I might have otherwise enjoyed if I'd been properly prepared for it (*Trainspotting*, as it turns out, was not quite the ode to railways that I was hoping for . . .).

So that's what this introduction is about: setting expectations. Perhaps I should start with a bit of background. I've always enjoyed eating but, until a few years ago, I'd never really thought very deeply about my diet. Which is not to say that I'd never really worried about my diet: like most people I was constantly watching my weight and stressed about whether or not I was eating the right foods or the right amount of food. But at some point I realized that I didn't need to live with that uncertainty. Like any physical system, the body is governed by rules that determine how different inputs – for example, diets – are transformed into different outputs – for example, health. To eliminate the stress associated with eating, I simply needed to learn the rules that determine how diet affects health and then use those rules to make systematic choices about what I eat.

Easier said than done, right? It's true that the rules that determine how diet affects health are complicated but they're not actually *that* complicated. They only seem complicated when you try to infer them from the information that you get through mass media. Much of the information about diet and health in mass media is, of course, exaggerated if not altogether incorrect but, even if it were accurate, the piecemeal nature of it would still be a major problem. The different systems in the body and brain that link diet and health are highly interdependent, so it's impossible to understand how some of them work without understanding how all of them work.

There is only one way to eliminate the uncertainty associated with eating: comprehensive understanding of the relevant science. I could give you a list of good and bad foods today but, even if you trusted me completely, just knowing that a particular food was considered to be good without understanding why wouldn't resolve your uncertainty. What if you saw a headline tomorrow demonizing that food? Would you then move that food to the bad list, only to move it back to the good list again when, inevitably, you saw a different headline the next day canonizing it?

And, of course, the idea that foods are either good or bad is overly simplistic. Take red meat for example: it's very nutritious, i.e. it contains a lot of important nutrients beyond those that are used directly for energy, like protein, vitamins and minerals, some of which can be difficult to obtain from other sources. But red meat has also repeatedly been linked to cardiovascular disease and cancer, and recent studies have identified the biological basis of these links. So where does that leave you? Is red meat good or bad? Do the benefits outweigh the risks or vice versa?

It may seem like I'm coming on a bit strong but I need you to buy into the idea that, when it comes to healthy eating, superficiality is not going to cut it. In fact, superficiality is exactly what got us into the mess that we're in today. Any attempt to make systematic choices about what you eat based on superficial understanding will only end in one way: confusion (which, of course, works out well for the nutritional-media-industrial complex because it keeps you continually clicking on their articles and buying their products, but that's a topic for another time...). The only way to keep your head from spinning in the midst of all the noise from mass media is to be confident enough in your understanding to ignore it.

If you want to solve the problem of eating once and for all, then you need to understand things well enough to answer any practical question correctly and confidently. If you are considering a change in your diet, you need to be able to marshal the relevant facts (and, therefore, be able to distinguish facts, i.e. conclusions from trustworthy experiments, from non-facts, i.e. everything else) and use them, along with knowledge of how all of the relevant systems in the body and brain interact, to predict what consequences, if any, that change in diet will have on your health. Achieving that level of understanding may be a tall order but it is certainly doable. Unlike much of science, where it seems that the more we know the less we understand, eating actually turns out to be relatively simple at the level of detail that matters in practice. But, again, it's not enough for me to simply tell you that: if you want to be able to move forward without constantly second-guessing yourself, you need to go through the process of deriving that conclusion for yourself.

That's what I did. I dove into the scientific literature to learn everything I needed to know about the different systems that are related to eating. I was a bit worried because I was aware that nutritional science had often been criticized for the poor quality of its research. I found that some of this criticism was fair in that studies of human nutrition are often poorly designed. But many of the studies that use animals are, in fact, excellent and it was the results of these animal studies that I was after. Human studies are, of course, critical for empirical validation of the rules that determine how diet affects health. However, only animal studies can actually identify those rules in the first place because only animal experiments allow for the precise measurements and total control that are required to study biology in detail. In other words, well-designed human studies may provide an indication of whether a particular food is ultimately good or bad but only animal studies can determine why.

So I read a few hundred studies, human and animal, and learned everything I needed to know related to diet and health. Using the understanding that I derived from the animal studies, I was able to correctly predict the results of the human studies without any apparent inconsistencies or contradictions in my reasoning. This was very exciting; I understood eating! I felt empowered by the knowledge that I would never again be stressed because of uncertainty about how my diet would affect my health. From now on, I would be able to choose my foods to achieve whatever combination of enjoyment and health I thought was most appropriate. But I soon realized that I'd only solved part of the problem and it was the easy part.

I suppose it's obvious in retrospect but while understanding the benefits and risks associated with different foods is definitely necessary, it's not sufficient. Like many people, I often found myself eating bad foods that I hadn't planned to eat and continuing to do so anyway. The real challenge when it comes to staying healthy isn't knowing which foods to eat, it's actually eating those foods. But I was not deterred. There was no reason why the same systematic approach wouldn't work again. Hunger isn't random. Nor is it controlled by the whim of some unknowable power. It is an output generated by a physical system according to a set of rules. If I wanted to control my hunger, rather than let it control me, I simply needed to learn those rules and then manipulate the relevant factors to achieve the desired output (this may sound brash but it is also true).

So I dove back into the scientific literature. This time I had a head start; through my work as a neuroscientist I was already familiar with the basic functions of the different brain regions that are involved in the control of hunger. But there was still plenty more to learn, so I read another few hundred studies – again, human and animal – to learn everything I needed to know about hunger. I'd already understood the rules that determine how diet affects health. That understanding allowed me to make systematic decisions about which foods to eat but it didn't tell me what I needed to do to make sure that I actually ate them. Now I also understood the rules that determine how lifestyle and environment affect hunger and, therefore, diet. So, by putting the old rules and the new rules together, I had the comprehensive understanding that I needed to give me full control over my eating.

And it works! For several years now, my diet has brought me great pleasure and kept me healthy, without any uncertainty or stress. I almost never eat unplanned snacks or overeat at planned meals. But it's not because I possess superhuman willpower; in fact, it's quite the opposite. I don't need any willpower because I've figured out how to adapt my lifestyle and my environment so that my hunger is directed towards the right foods at the right times. And, just to be clear, I do not eat exclusively good foods: eating bad foods is actually a source of great enjoyment for me. That's the power of actually understanding eating: I don't have to err on the side of caution just to be sure that I remain healthy. Instead, I'm able to enjoy eating as much as I possibly can without compromising my health.

So I'd figured out how to take total control of my eating but it was an awful lot of effort. I decided to write this book to make it more convenient for others to do the same. It's really totally unacceptable that eating is a cause of ill health and unhappiness for so many people. I see it as nothing less than a fundamental failure of our society. And while I would love to believe that the organizations with the power to facilitate large-scale changes in the way we eat will finally acknowledge the true nature of the problem and act accordingly, I'm not holding my breath. It would be naive to hope for significant policy changes in the short term (and even more naive, of course, to hope that processed food manufacturers suddenly suffer a crisis of conscience and impose change on themselves).

The sad thing is that healthy eating, at least in terms of the biology, is a solved problem. You might think that we still have a lot to learn but we don't, at least not at the level of detail that matters in practice. We know which foods are healthy and which foods aren't and we know what causes people to choose the latter over the former. What we don't yet know, however, is how to overcome the many challenges that prevent healthy eating from being the norm, some of which are real – for example, the logistical problems associated with making unprocessed foods available to everyone – and some of which are simply obstacles created by those who profit either directly or indirectly from unhealthy eating (but that's yet another topic for another time…). The approach that worked for me – building a comprehensive understanding of eating and using it to derive personal solutions – may not be practical for everyone but I'm confident that it will work for a lot of people. And at the moment, it's really the only option.

So anyway, that's the background, now let's get back to setting expectations. Developing a comprehensive understanding of something as complex as eating is not easy: it requires detailed knowledge of concepts from many different scientific fields ranging from molecular biology to psychology, as well as background knowledge of other areas like evolution, statistics and scientific methodology. As I was developing my understanding, I had to keep going back and forth between many different research studies to identify where my understanding was failing and to learn what I needed to eliminate those failures. If you want to understand eating well enough to take full control of your diet and your health, you have no choice but to go through the same process of developing and refining your understanding for yourself. But this book will make that process a lot easier.

Part of the book's value is simply that it eliminates the need to consult multiple sources; all of the information that you need is right here in one place. The book also presents the information in the optimal order, which makes everything a lot easier. The trick when trying to develop a comprehensive understanding of something complex is to minimize the number of inconsistencies and large knowledge gaps that need to be resolved along the way, so the ordering of the information can make a big difference. But the book does much more than simply provide all of the relevant information in the appropriate order: it also presents the information in a format that is easy to parse and integrate into your understanding.

The book is written in casual language rather than the complex, jargon-filled sentences that are typically used in scientific writing. But please don't mistake this lack of formality for a lack of seriousness (I hope that by now you're convinced that I take eating very seriously…). Any idea, no matter how complex, can be expressed perfectly well in plain language without "dumbing it down." The dense and esoteric nature of traditional scientific writing may have some advantages for communication between experts but it is certainly not a prerequisite for high-level discourse.

In addition to casual language, the book uses a very non-traditional structure involving a dialogue between two people rather than standard prose. This format may take some getting used to but I chose it very deliberately because it has distinct advantages. The dialogue format allows the flow of information to be carefully controlled so that each new piece can be integrated and reconciled with those that came before it in a way that would be difficult with standard prose. The conversation between the two people in the book is essentially the conversation that I had with myself as I was developing my own understanding. By observing the process by which I integrated each new piece of information into my understanding and how I identified potential inconsistencies and contradictions as they arose and reconciled them before moving on, it will be much easier for you to replicate the process yourself.

Finally, there is one other advantage to the dialogue format: it forces you to actually read the book. The dialogue format precludes skimming or dipping in and out; there is no way to read this book other than concentrating and going line-by-line. I admit that it may be a bit presumptuous for me to be telling you how to read but you have to keep in mind the purpose of the book. If you really want to develop a comprehensive and detailed understanding of something as complex as eating, then I'm sorry but you're going to have to concentrate!

If you're willing to invest a few hours of attentive reading, you'll learn everything you need to be able to take control of your eating and make yourself healthier and happier for the rest of your life. That's a pretty good deal! So wait until you know you're going to have some large chunks of time to spare over the course of a week or two and then settle in and power through. Don't get discouraged if you don't understand everything right away; the same concepts will keep coming up again and again. And don't be satisfied with anything less than complete understanding. I promise you that the book contains all of the information that you need or at least nearly all of it: the understanding developed in the book is sort of generic, so it's possible that you may want a bit more information about certain aspects of eating that are especially relevant for you.

And while we're talking about the understanding that the book will help you develop, let me take a moment to clarify its nature. Some readers might be hoping for a quantitative model, i.e. a set of equations that describes the interactions between all of the relevant variables and predicts precise output values along with measures of confidence in those predictions. Wouldn't it be great if there was a model into which you could plug in exactly what you planned to eat and get out exactly how your weight and health would change as a result? Forget it. The science of eating is not yet far enough along to allow the development of such a model; in fact, it's not even close. But that's OK, because you don't need a quantitative model to take control of your eating.

There are situations where quantitative models are critical – like, say, weather prediction, where a tiny change in one input can lead to large, complex changes in outputs. Fortunately, eating isn't like that. At the practical level that is relevant for choosing what to eat, the relationship between diet and health is very simple. For a huge range of inputs, i.e. diets, the outputs are exactly the same: stable body weight and good health (this is one of the many reasons why the confusion created by the noise in mass media is such a shame: very little of what is discussed actually matters). And even when things get outside the healthy range, the changes are very stereotyped. There is no point in trying to predict the small fluctuations in weight and health that may occur within the healthy range (even if you could, why would you want to?). We simply need to make sure that we do what is needed to stay within that range or what is needed to get ourselves back into it if we have left it, and for that purpose a semi-quantitative or even a qualitative understanding is perfectly sufficient.

Let me also say that the book doesn't provide the details of every relevant biochemical pathway. Again, this is because that level of detail is not relevant for practical purposes. The details that are needed for practical purposes are complex enough as it is, so I don't see any point in including more. For example, it's important that you know that there are gut bacteria that convert a chemical in red meat into a different chemical that can encourage the build-up of plaques in your blood vessels. It isn't, however, important that you know the name of those bacteria, the name of those chemicals or the details of the process by which those bacteria perform the conversion. And if you do decide that you do want more details than I've provided, you can always read the research studies yourself.

Which leads me to my last point: there don't seem to be any agreed-upon standards for referencing in a book like this, so I've done what I think makes the most sense. When I make a quantitative statement or semi-quantitative statement, I cite the original research study or studies on which the statement is based, e.g. "One in four adults in the US has fatty liver disease" or "most people who lose weight just end up regaining it." When I describe the results of a study or group of studies in detail, I cite the studies when I first begin to describe them, e.g. "Let's start with what we know from experiments with cells in a dish."

And, finally, when I provide background information on a particular topic, I cite one or several review papers that provide a good overview of the state-of-the-art in that topic, e.g. "Maybe I should explain a little bit about how the stress system works" or "Fiber fat is really important." In the event that there are multiple reviews that are equally comprehensive and authoritative, I cite those that I believe to be the most accessible to non-experts.

OK? Good: then if you're ready, let's get started.

Introduction II

Whoa, he's back from the dead!

Oh, c'mon.

Seriously, I haven't seen you for ages. How are you?

I'm good. How are you?

I'm fine. What have you been up to? Busy with work?

Sort of. Actually, I've been working on a book.

Oh, cool. You're a neuroscientist right? Is it a book about the brain?

No. Well, kind of. It's really about eating.

Eating? How'd you get into that?

I don't know, I've kind of always been into food.

Oh, I didn't know you were a foodie.

Well, I don't know if I'm a foodie but I certainly enjoy eating.

So is it a cookbook with all of your favorite recipes?

No, no. It's about the science of eating: diet, metabolism, stuff like that. I was seeing all of these newspaper articles that were making my head spin – you know, one day something is good for you and the next day it's not. I guess I figured it was time I sorted it out for myself.

Is there really that much to know?

Are you kidding? Do you have any idea what happens to food after you swallow it?

Not really. But does it matter?

Well, how do you decide what to eat?

I don't know. I just try to eat mostly healthy stuff and allow myself an unhealthy treat now and then.

But how do you know what's healthy and what's unhealthy?

Is it really that complicated? Fruits and vegetables are healthy, fast food and sweets are unhealthy and so on.

OK, first of all, I guarantee that many of the foods that you think are unhealthy are actually healthy and vice versa. And, second of all, if everyone knows what they should and shouldn't be eating, then why are so many people overweight?

Because they eat unhealthy foods, even though they know they shouldn't. And I guess they also don't exercise enough.

OK, well, again, I think there are many people who have the wrong idea about which foods are healthy and unhealthy. But there are also a lot of people who have the right idea and are trying to be healthy but failing. Most overweight people try to lose weight and fail again and again. Now, maybe some of those people only make a half-hearted attempt at it but many of them do really believe that their situation is unhealthy and they desperately try to lose weight but still fail. Don't you find that strange? Do you really just want to blame that on a lack of willpower?

Well, what else can it be?

It's complicated. Do you have any idea why you get hungry when you do?

I guess it's because I'm low on energy.

No. Even lean people always have enough energy to go for days without food. Overweight people could go for weeks. What do you think body fat is? It's stored energy.

OK, so why do overweight people ever get hungry?

Well, that's a great question. The fact that they do should tell you that the whole thing is not as simple as you might think.

OK, so is this where your book comes in?

Yeah, sort of. When I started looking for a book that covered all of the relevant science, I realized there wasn't one.

What about a text book?

That's where I started, and I found a couple of good ones but the problem is that text books are sometimes a decade or two behind. And when it comes to eating, that's a real problem, because we've learned a lot in recent years.

But don't people write books about eating all the time? There must be a few out there that are pretty good.

You're right, there are. I've read a lot of them and many of them are good but they all seem to have a particular focus. They usually have one message like "Sugar is bad" or "Fat is good," but they never give you the whole picture.

So you pieced it all together from reading a lot of different books?

No, in the end I had to go back and read all the original research studies. The whole thing turned out to be *a lot* more complicated that I thought.

How so?

Well, I guess I thought that if I understood the biology of digestion and metabolism, that would get me most of the way. But there's actually much more to it than that.

Like what?

Like the brain, for starters. Healthy eating is ultimately about decision making and obviously that involves the brain. But I suppose that's not too surprising. The real surprises were the role of the immune system and the role of gut bacteria.

What do they have to do with eating?

Oh, everything. They're incredibly important.

Really?

Really. To be honest, I think the two most important advances in all of science in recent years are related to the immune system and gut bacteria. It's no surprise that the immune system is important in general but we now know that all of the bad things that happen when you're overweight – diabetes, heart attacks, strokes and so on – aren't really caused by excess body fat itself, they're caused by the way your immune system responds to excess body fat.

Wow. And what about gut bacteria?

Oh, gut bacteria are really the next great frontier in biology and medicine. They're this century's DNA. Over the past decade, we've learned that gut bacteria are critical to every aspect of health but especially digestion and metabolism. There is still a lot more to learn but it's already clear that gut bacteria are incredibly important.

Man, you're fired up! So your book lays this all out?

That's right.

Can you run me through it?

I guess so, but it could take a while.

I've got time…

1
Metabolism

Energy

OK, well, before we can get into any of the really interesting stuff, there are a few basic things that you need to understand. I guess we should start with metabolism. Your metabolic systems keep all of the different parts of your body supplied with energy. Because you only eat a few times per day, you need systems that store extra energy after eating and release it slowly between meals.

OK, that sounds simple enough.

Well, there are a few details to consider. First of all, you use two different sources of energy: glucose, which comes from carbohydrates, and fat, which comes from, well, fat. Your muscles – and most of the rest of the cells in your body – are happy to use either but your brain isn't. Your brain uses only glucose.

Why doesn't my brain use fat?

Because fat has trouble getting into your brain. Glucose and fat are transported around your body in your blood. Your blood generally moves freely around your body but to enter your brain it has to pass through a filter called the blood-brain barrier. This filter keeps a lot of things out to protect your brain. It turns out that glucose can get through the filter easily but fat can't.

OK. But if my body and brain are both happy to use glucose, then why don't I just stick to that and give up on fat altogether?

Good question. The problem is that glucose doesn't store very well; it's hard to pack together and it takes up a lot of space. Fat, on the other hand, packs together really well, so it's perfect for storage.

I see. OK. I guess if most of my body is happy to use fat, and it can be stored more efficiently than glucose, then it makes sense to store most of my energy as fat.

Right. That's what your fat cells are: storage containers for fat.

But I must need to store at least some glucose to keep my brain going if I don't eat?

Yes, that's right, you do store a bit of glucose in your liver, which is your main metabolic organ.

I only store a bit of glucose? That seems risky. What if I don't eat for a while?

Exactly. If you have to go for a while without eating any glucose, you need a backup plan.[1]

Right. So what is it?

Your liver doesn't just store glucose, it also makes it whenever your body or brain need it.

From what?

Mostly from the waste that is created when you use glucose and fat for energy.

Oh, that's clever. It's like recycling.

Right.

OK, I take it back, this is getting complicated.

Don't worry, we'll keep coming back to these basic concepts over and over again. This will all be second nature to you by the end, I promise. Why don't you try to summarize what I've told you so far?

OK. For energy sources, I've got glucose and fat coming in from food, and glucose being made in my liver.

Right.

For energy storage, I've got my liver storing glucose and my fat cells storing fat.

Right.

And for energy use, I've got my brain using only glucose and my muscles using either glucose or fat.

Good. So let's assume you've just woken up in the morning. What's happening?

Well, I haven't eaten in a while, so all of my energy must be coming from storage. My liver is sending glucose to my brain and my fat cells are sending fat to my muscles.

Right. Now what happens when you eat?

Well, I guess some of the glucose from the food will be used by my brain and the rest will be stored in my liver. And some of the fat from the food will be used by my muscles and the rest will be stored in my fat cells.

That's close. But, remember, you can't store that much glucose.

Right. But if I eat a lot of glucose, my muscles can just use that instead of fat for a while.

Exactly.

Well that's not that bad, then. The only question is whether my muscles are going to use glucose or fat after a meal and that just depends on how much glucose I've just eaten.

Insulin

Right, so in the end, the basics are pretty simple. But the whole thing needs to be regulated. You need a system that makes sure that the glucose and fat from each meal are sent to the right places.

That doesn't sound too complicated.

Sure, the concept is simple, but how are you actually going to do it?

Well, I guess the glucose and fat that I eat all enters my blood in the same place...

That's right, in your intestines.

OK, so I just need something near my intestines that tracks what's coming in.

Yes, that's exactly what your pancreas does. But how do you then get the glucose and fat where they need to go?

Oh, I see the problem. My blood goes everywhere in my body, so I can't just send the glucose to one part of my body and the fat to another.

Right.

OK, OK, let's see. If the glucose and fat are going everywhere then maybe each part of my body decides for itself what to take out of my blood?

Or each part of your body could be told what to take out of your blood...

I see. So my pancreas, which is keeping track of how much glucose and fat are coming in, is also telling different parts of my body whether they should be using glucose or fat?

That's right, and the signal your pancreas uses is insulin – that's your glucose hormone.

Sorry, what's a hormone?

Oh, sorry, I shouldn't use scientific terms without explaining them. You should definitely stop me when I do that. A hormone is a chemical that carries a message through your blood from one place to another.

OK. So as glucose comes into my blood, my pancreas releases insulin?

Right.

What about fat?

Your pancreas ignores fat.

Really? OK, so when I eat glucose, my pancreas releases insulin to tell my muscles that they should use glucose instead of fat.

Exactly.

How does it work?

Well, before you can understand how insulin works, you have to understand how glucose and fat get into your cells. You can't just have glucose and fat coming into cells whenever they want to, they have to be controlled. Glucose needs an escort to get into a cell and insulin activates the escort. Insulin goes into a cell, tells the escort that there is some glucose waiting outside and then the escort goes and brings the glucose into the cell.

OK.

So the amount of glucose that gets into your cells is controlled by the amount of insulin in your blood.

Got it.

Good. But we have to think about fat as well. The amount of fat coming into your cells is also controlled by insulin but less directly. Unlike glucose, fat can actually move in and out of cells without an escort.

So where is the control?

Insulin controls how much fat is in your blood.

How?

It tells your fat cells whether they should be storing or releasing fat.[2]

OK, let me see if I get it. After a meal with a lot of glucose, my pancreas will release insulin, which will tell my muscles to use glucose and my fat cells to store fat. Between meals, my pancreas will stop releasing insulin, so my fat cells will release fat into my blood and that fat will get used by my muscles.

Right. And don't forget about your liver.

Right. I guess insulin also tells my liver whether it should be storing or releasing glucose?

Exactly. After a meal with a lot of glucose, your insulin will be high, which will tell your liver to store glucose. Between meals, your insulin will be low, so your liver will release the glucose that it has stored and also any that it makes.

OK, I think I get it, but it's hard to keep it all straight. Let me try to sum it up.

Go ahead.

OK. When I wake up in the morning, my insulin is low, so my fat cells are releasing fat to be used by my muscles and my liver is releasing and making glucose to be used by my brain.

Right.

Then, when I eat breakfast, my insulin goes up, which tells my muscles to use glucose from the meal, tells my liver to store glucose from the meal and tells my fat cells to store fat from the meal.

Exactly! And the same cycle repeats throughout the day as you go from meal to meal.

Food

OK, I think I get everything you've said so far, but what about all the rest of the things in food? There's a lot more to food than just glucose and fat, right? What about protein and vitamins and all the rest of that stuff?

You're right. There are some other important things in food besides glucose and fat. Maybe we should take a step back for a minute and talk about food more generally?

OK.

OK. Anything you eat, whether it's a plant or an animal, is made up of some combination of proteins, vitamins, minerals, carbs and fat. All of those things are important but, if we're going to focus on metabolism and weight regulation, we don't really need to talk much about proteins and we can totally ignore vitamins and minerals, at least until the very end.

Really?

Protein can actually be used for energy but it's kind of a last resort. All of the protein in your body is there for some other purpose, so you don't really want to be using it for energy. You just need to make sure you eat enough of it. The same goes for vitamins and minerals. Now, don't get me wrong, there are *a lot* of people who don't get enough protein, vitamins or minerals and are unhealthy because of it. But, for the most part, those are people whose access to food is restricted because they're poor or because they live in a place where unprocessed food is hard to get. For you, it shouldn't be something you need to worry about: if you eat a reasonable variety of natural foods, you'll be fine. We'll get to the really big-picture diet stuff at the end, but it'll make more sense if you understand what's going on in your body first.

OK, so we're only worried about carbs and fat.

Right. Now, there are two kinds of carbs, the ones you can digest and the ones you can't. The carbs you can digest come in a few different basic forms. The most important are glucose, which we've already discussed, and fructose, which is the one that actually tastes sweet.

Glucose doesn't taste sweet?

No.

So sugar is fructose, not glucose?

I assume that by "sugar" you mean the white crystals that you put in your coffee or use for baking?

Right.

That is half glucose and half fructose.

Oh, OK.

And that's really the only way you'll ever find fructose: in combination with glucose as sugar. Glucose, on the other hand, also comes in large strings on its own, called starches. Things like white bread, white rice and pasta are just long strings of glucose.

OK, so when we eat carbs, we're really just eating either long strings of glucose or little pairs of glucose and fructose?

That's right, if you're thinking about only the carbs you can digest.

Right. Wait, if we can digest fructose but it's not used for energy, what is it used for?

Ah, now that is a very important question. Thousands of years ago, our ancestors wouldn't have eaten that much sugar, so it wouldn't have mattered that much. There is sugar in many natural foods like fruits but the amounts are relatively small. But now that we've started extracting sugar from plants and adding it to everything, we're eating much more of it than we used to. So the question of what happens to fructose when it enters your body has suddenly become very important. We'll get into the details of that in a minute but I think it would be better to finish talking about food first.

OK, go on.

OK, so there are also carbs that you can't digest called fiber.

So what happens when we eat fiber, it just passes right through?

Well, no. Actually, fiber does get digested – not by you but by your gut bacteria.

What?

Listen, I know you're going to have a lot of questions as we go along. I'll try to answer some of them, especially if you just need

clarification, but I need you to try to go with the flow and trust me. There is a lot you need to know and I'm trying to tell you things in the order that will make it easiest for you to see the whole picture in the end. I promise I will answer all of your questions eventually.

OK, sorry, go on.

Right, so the different kinds of carbs you need to think about are glucose, fructose and fiber. There are also different kinds of fat.

Right, I know that there are good and bad fats.

Yes, I suppose there are, although you're probably thinking of good and bad fats in terms of how they affect your cholesterol. It turns out that was all wrong.

Really? Wait, what is cholesterol anyway? Is that a kind of fat?

Yes, but it's not used for energy. It is used by your cells for a lot of other important things though. There is cholesterol in food but we're not going to worry about it.

Why not?

Because you actually make a lot of cholesterol yourself. If you eat more of it, your body will make less. If you eat less of it, your body will make more. Either way, the amount of cholesterol in your body will stay pretty much the same.[3]

Really? OK...

Don't worry, we'll talk a lot about cholesterol later. First, let's get back to the different kinds of fats. Actually, you know what? The distinction between different fats isn't going to make any sense until later when we start talking about inflammation. I think we can go through digestion and a few other things without worrying about that.

OK.

Good, so when it comes to food, we've only got four things to worry about. There are starches, like pasta, rice and bread, which are long strings of glucose.

Right.

There's sugar, which is a combination of glucose and fructose.

Right.

There's fiber, which is the part of plants that we can't digest.

Right.

And there are fats, which we're just grouping all together for now.

Got it.

Digestion

Good, then let's move on to digestion. The first thing you do when you digest food is to break it down into its basic units. You break starches into glucose, you break sugar into glucose and fructose and you break fats into their basic unit, which is called a fatty acid. You start by chewing, which breaks food into smaller pieces. Then you swallow and pass the small pieces of food to your stomach.

What about saliva, is that just to lubricate things?

Mostly. There are actually some enzymes in saliva that can break down carbs.

OK. Wait, what's an enzyme?

Oh, an enzyme is just something that causes a chemical reaction. The important thing about enzymes is that they're very specific. So the enzymes in saliva break down carbs but they have no effect on fat or anything else.

OK. Go on.

As small pieces of food arrive in your stomach, your stomach breaks them down into even smaller pieces and also adds in some acid and some more enzymes to help things along. So now you've got a half-digested mush. Your stomach passes this mush into your intestines, where it finally gets broken down all the way and passed into your blood.

Except for the fiber.

That's right. We'll talk a lot about fiber later but let's not worry about it for now. Let's talk about what happens to the other carbs and fats in your intestine. Starches and sugar are broken down all the way into glucose and fructose, and fats are broken down all the way into fatty acids. The glucose and fructose go straight into your blood as they are but the fatty acids are actually regrouped into bigger packages together with some other stuff, including cholesterol.

Why?

Because glucose and fructose will move around nicely in your blood on their own but fat won't. If you put fat into your blood alone, it will just all clump together. So most of the fat in your blood is transported around in packages together with cholesterol. This is actually a really important point. There are a few different kinds of these fat packages and the differences between them determine, for example, how likely they are to get stuck in your blood vessels. But we'll get to all that in a minute.

OK, so what I need to know so far is that glucose and fructose are sent straight into my blood but fatty acids are packaged together first.

Right, let's just call those "digested fat packages."

Do they have another name?

Yes, but it's horrible. I really think that we should avoid using scientific jargon whenever we can. We've got *a lot* of complicated concepts to cover and I don't see any point in making them even more complicated by introducing new terms if we don't need to. If something is really important and we're going to talk about it a lot, like insulin, then we can use the scientific term. Otherwise, let's just use terms that make sense.

OK, well, if you think I'm too dumb to use the scientific terms, then I guess we shouldn't use them…

Oh, c'mon, that's not it at all. I'm not talking to you any differently than I would talk to another scientist. It's true that scientific writing can be hard to understand, but when scientists actually talk to each other in person, this is how they talk, in plain language. And, anyway, I don't see why you would be offended by someone who is trying to explain things as clearly as possible. What I would be offended by is someone who was too lazy or pompous to bother.

OK, OK, go on.

The liver

OK, so all of the stuff from your intestine – the glucose, the fructose and the digested fat packages – are passed into your blood and pumped straight into your liver. We already know what happens to the glucose.

Right. Some gets stored and the rest just passes through.

Right. And the digested fat packages just pass right through.

OK.

Now what happens to fructose in your liver is really important. Your liver actually does *a lot* more than just store and make glucose. Your liver is the only place in your body where fructose can be processed.

Wait, let me guess. My liver converts fructose into glucose?

That's a good guess, especially given what I've told you so far. And, in fact, you're right. Your liver can convert fructose into glucose and it might actually do it if there isn't a lot of glucose already around. But you really only eat fructose together with glucose as sugar and usually with a lot more glucose as starches as well. What I haven't told you yet is that your liver can also make fat.

Uh oh. OK, I see where this is going.

Well, that doesn't need to be a bad thing. Like with glucose, your liver normally makes fat from the waste that is created when glucose and fat are used for energy, so, again, it's a form of recycling. Your liver will package the fat that it makes together with cholesterol, which it also makes, and release the packages into your blood. As I said, cholesterol is used by your cells for all kinds of important things. So under normal conditions, the fact that your liver is making and releasing fat packages is a good thing.

OK. You said that digested fats are also packed together with cholesterol, so are liver fat packages and digested fat packages the same?

Yes and no. They are the same in that they both contain fat and cholesterol but they are different in size, and this turns out to be really important.

OK, hold on, I want to make sure I've got it all straight.

Go ahead.

After a meal, I've got glucose, fructose and digested fat packages coming from my intestines into my blood and through my liver.

Right.

Some of the glucose is stored in my liver for later and the rest passes through to be used for energy right away by my muscles and brain.

Right.

The digested fat packages pass straight through my liver and I guess my fat cells pick them up for storage?

Right.

OK. And my liver converts the fructose into fat, packages it and releases it into my blood. I guess the fat packages from my liver get picked up by my fat cells as well?

That's right.

Summary I

OK, why don't you try to run me through the whole thing? So you just ate a big meal, what happens?

OK. My mouth, stomach and intestines break everything down into its basic units: starches into glucose, sugar into glucose and fructose, and fats into fatty acids.

Right.

The fatty acids get regrouped together with cholesterol into digested fat packages and then everything goes from my intestines into my blood.

Right.

My pancreas sees the glucose and releases insulin.

Right.

My liver stores some of the glucose and makes and releases fat packages from the fructose.

Right.

My fat cells store fat from the digested and liver fat packages.

Right.

And my brain and muscles use the rest of the glucose.

Excellent! And now, between meals, what happens?

My pancreas stops releasing insulin.

Right.

My liver starts making and releasing glucose.

Right.

My fat cells start releasing fat.

Right.

My brain keeps using glucose.

Right.

And my muscles switch to using fat.

Outstanding! That's it. Those are the basics of metabolism.

OK, can I ask a couple of questions now?

Please do; go ahead.

2
Inflammation

Fructose

OK, I think I'm good with glucose, that seems pretty straightforward. But fructose I'm less sure about. You seem to be implying that fructose is particularly bad and I don't see why. If it gets converted to fat, why is it any different than just eating fat?

Good question. The conversion of fructose to fat is particularly bad for a couple of reasons. First of all, processing fructose is actually bad for your liver.[1] It can handle small amounts without too much trouble but forcing your liver to process fructose constantly is going to cause serious damage. In fact, your liver processes fructose the same way as it processes alcohol, so all of the liver problems that can be caused by alcohol can also be caused by fructose.

Really?

Sure. As far as your liver is concerned, soda and beer are basically the same.

Hold on. I know a lot of people who drink a lot of soda and they don't all have liver problems.

Yes they do! Something like one in four adults in the US have fatty liver disease.[2]

What's that?

It's when you start storing a lot of fat in your liver. Your liver can only make and release fat packages at a certain rate so if you eat too much fructose and it gets converted to fat faster than your liver

can package and release it, then it will end up getting stored in your liver instead. And your liver isn't really meant to store fat so, when it does, it stops working properly. Having too much fat in your liver is a really big deal, because it changes the fat packages that your liver releases.

Fat packages

Right, the whole fat-packaged-with-cholesterol thing is still a little confusing; I've got a few questions about that. First of all, what about the fat that is released from my fat cells between meals? Is that packaged as well?

Oh, sorry, I wasn't clear about that. The fat released from your fat cells isn't packaged with cholesterol, it's just fatty acids.

But you said that fat won't move around nicely in my blood on its own. Isn't that the whole point of the digested fat packages and liver fat packages?

Yes, you're right. In fact, the fatty acids released from your fat cells are also in a kind of package, but it's a very simple package and the only important thing inside it is the fatty acids. The fat released from your fat cells is meant to be used for energy right away, so the packaging is really the bare minimum. I think it's safe to ignore it and just think of your fat cells as releasing fatty acids.

OK, so in terms of fat in my blood, I've got digested fat packages and liver fat packages, both of which also contain cholesterol, and fatty acids from my fat cells.

Right. I think we're ready to talk more about cholesterol.

OK, good.

Remember, cholesterol is also a fat and, even though it isn't used for energy, it still needs to be sent to your cells, so it travels together with fatty acids in the digested fat packages and the liver fat packages.

OK.

Now, as the fat and cholesterol are removed from the packages and used by your cells, waste is created. This waste is picked up by other packages and taken back to your liver for recycling. Let's call those "waste packages."

OK.

And after most of the fat and cholesterol have been removed from the digested and liver fat packages, the mostly empty packages also find their way back to your liver. Let's call those "depleted packages."

OK. So then, in my liver, the waste from the waste packages and the depleted digested fat packages and depleted liver fat packages are all recycled to make more fat, more cholesterol and more liver fat packages?

Right.

Fine. I really don't see how cholesterol becomes a problem. You've said that it's used for important things and that my body makes sure that I have the same amount of cholesterol in my blood no matter what I eat. What's the problem?

Good question. I think we're through most of the basics now, so we can start to talk about what happens when things go wrong. Why don't you try to summarize the different fat packages for me again first?

OK. There are digested fat packages and liver fat packages, which contain fatty acids and cholesterol.

Right.

There are fatty acids from fat cells, which are in a simple package we're ignoring.

Right.

And there are waste packages that take waste from cells that are using fat and cholesterol.

Right. And don't forget the depleted digested and liver fat packages, those are really important.

Right, OK, got it.

Obesity

OK. So far, so good, right? Your body has metabolic systems that allow you to use, store and even make glucose and fat, with most of your cells able to use either depending on what's available. Yet most people are overweight or obese, at least in developed countries,[3] so something is clearly not working.

Right, so what's going wrong?

OK, so here is one of the main themes that will keep coming up throughout our whole discussion: one of the biggest reasons that most people struggle to control their weight is that there is a huge mismatch between the environment that we evolved in and the environment that we live in today.[4]

What do you mean?

The foods that we eat today are very different from what our ancestors used to eat. First of all, the processed foods that we eat today are much easier to digest.

Sorry, but what exactly are processed foods?

Well, I suppose processed foods are foods that have been altered by humans in any way at all. We'll talk about a lot of different types of food processing eventually, but there are really two main types of processing that we need to worry about: removing fiber and adding sugar. Let's talk about removing fiber first.

OK.

In natural, unprocessed foods, glucose is surrounded by fiber, so it takes a while for your intestines to sort everything out. But in processed foods, like white bread and white rice, the fiber has been removed, so you can digest the glucose really quickly.

So the glucose from processed foods gets into my blood much faster than the glucose from unprocessed foods?

That's right.

OK. So what?

Well, for your metabolism to work properly, your pancreas has to match the amount of insulin it releases to the amount of glucose that you eat. But it can't do that accurately when a lot of glucose comes into your blood at once.

Why not?

Well, until recently, it didn't have to. For millions of years, animals and, eventually, humans ate only unprocessed foods and our metabolic systems evolved accordingly.

OK. So when I eat processed foods and the glucose comes into my blood too quickly, my pancreas doesn't release enough insulin?

No, actually it's the opposite. When too much glucose comes into your blood too quickly, your pancreas overreacts and releases too much insulin.

Oh, OK. And why is that bad?

Why don't you tell me?

Well, when my pancreas releases insulin, my muscles switch to using glucose for energy, my fat cells start storing fat and my liver starts storing glucose.

Right.

So, I guess if my pancreas releases too much insulin, the glucose in my blood will get used up but my fat cells and liver won't start releasing anything because there will still be a lot of insulin in my blood.

Exactly.

OK, so if I eat a lot of processed foods that are easy to digest and my pancreas releases too much insulin, I'll end up with low blood glucose and low blood fat.[5] That doesn't sound good.

Well, it's no big deal if it happens once in a while. But if you're always eating processed foods, you'll have a lot of these insulin overshoots and that's when the trouble starts. We'll talk a lot more about this later but, basically, if your blood glucose and fat get too low, your brain will think that you are low on energy, so it will make you feel hungry and tired.[6] And, in a sense, you *are* low on energy. But it's not because you haven't eaten enough, it's because your fat cells and liver just keep storing energy when they should be releasing it.

OK, OK. So you're saying that people become obese because of a sort of vicious cycle in which they eat too much processed food, which causes an insulin overshoot, which leads to low blood glucose and low blood fat, which makes them hungry and tired and causes them to overeat again, and so on.[7]

Oh, no, the insulin overshoot is only one small part of the problem.

Really?

Yeah, we're just getting started. So let's say that you're starting to gain weight because you're eating too many processed foods. This is when the real trouble starts, because your immune system gets involved.

Uh oh.

Uh oh is right.

Inflammation

OK, so you probably already know that your immune system is your body's defence against infections, right?

Sure.

Good. So your immune cells are generally on patrol throughout your body and, if they detect something that isn't supposed to be there, they take action. There are quite a few things that immune cells can do, like release chemicals or swallow things.

OK.

But what's important for weight regulation is that your immune cells don't only take action against intruders: they also take action when things go wrong inside your body, for maintenance purposes.

Such as?

Such as when a cell dies or starts behaving strangely.

OK.

Good. Now, when your immune cells take action, that's called inflammation.

OK.

And inflammation is a good thing, until it's not. As I said earlier, it turns out that all of the unhealthy consequences of being over-weight – diabetes, heart attacks, strokes and so on – are caused by inflammation in excess body fat.

Really?

Really. Once you've gained so much weight that your body fat becomes inflamed, it kicks off a whole series of events that make you sick and make it really, really hard for you to ever lose the weight.

OK, I'm willing to believe that inflammation is important but I feel like you must be exaggerating a bit. I mean, why haven't I heard about this before?

I don't know. I understand your skepticism, though. We've known for a while that fat can become inflamed but it's really only recently, maybe in the last decade or so, that we've learned why that's such a problem.[8]

OK, please go on.

Insulin resistance and diabetes

OK, so one thing that really gets your immune system going is a build-up of waste in cells that are using or storing glucose or fat. If your cells get overwhelmed and can't process everything fast enough, things can get a bit messy.

What do you mean?

If your cells can't handle all of the glucose or fat that's coming into them, you'll end up with a lot of half-processed glucose and fat and a lot of waste.[9]

I see.

And if an immune cell notices this build-up, it will do what it can to help your cells catch up. For example, you remember that glucose needs an escort to enter a cell, right?

Right.

So, to prevent glucose from getting into your cells, your immune cells can release chemicals that interfere with that escort. Hopefully, that will slow things down enough for your cells to process their backlog of glucose and get things back to normal.

OK.

The same thing can happen with too much fat. If your fat cells are getting more fat than they can store, your immune cells will step in. They'll try to prevent fat from entering your fat cells and try to help release some of the fat that is already stored. Now, do you remember what normally controls the entry of glucose into a cell?

Insulin.

And what tells fat cells whether they should be storing or releasing fat?

Also insulin.

That's right. So the response of your immune cells to too much glucose and fat is to interfere with your insulin. Again, this is no big deal if it happens once in a while but, if you're in this situation we've been talking about where you're constantly overeating and your fat cells are always storing fat, it's going to become a serious problem.

Because my immune cells are going to be constantly taking action and my insulin isn't going to work anymore?

Exactly. That's called insulin resistance and it's the main reason that being overweight is unhealthy.[10] The problem is that the whole thing can get out of control very quickly. For example, as your fat cells get bigger and bigger, some of them will end up being so far away from any blood vessels that they'll die because they don't get enough oxygen. And what happens when cells die?

More inflammation.

Right. By the time you're obese, nearly half of the cells in your body fat will be immune cells.[11] And the chemicals released by all of those immune cells will start leaking out of your fat into the rest of your body and interfering with the insulin everywhere.

OK, I see the problem.

Oh, it's about to get much worse. If your insulin isn't working, the glucose in your blood will have trouble getting into your cells, so it will stay in your blood and you'll always have high blood glucose. And the insulin resistance will affect your liver as well. Normally, insulin would tell your liver to store glucose but, if your insulin isn't working, your liver will just keep making and releasing glucose, which will make things even worse.

Is this how diabetes starts?

Exactly. Because your immune system is interfering with your insulin, your liver will think that your insulin is always low, so it'll constantly make and release glucose. But since none of that glucose will be able to get into your cells, it will just keep floating around in your blood – that's diabetes.[12]

Right – and that's different from the other kind of diabetes, right?

Right. They should really have completely different names. People who have "Type 1" diabetes have no insulin because they don't have a working pancreas. But when they inject insulin into their blood, it works just fine. People who have "Type 2" diabetes – the kind that you get from overeating – have a working pancreas but their insulin doesn't work because their immune cells are interfering with it. But, it's also possible for your pancreas to stop working even with Type 2 diabetes. If your blood glucose is always high, your pancreas will just keep producing more and more insulin and, eventually, it will burn out.

I see.

Plaques, cholesterol, heart attacks and strokes

Good. And, don't forget, your fat cells will be releasing fat all of the time because of the insulin resistance, so you'll have high blood fat as well.

But at least I'll start losing weight then, right?

Not really. You might use some of the fat from your fat cells for energy but most of it will just float around in your blood until it gets picked up by your liver and put into liver fat packages. And that can cause serious problems.

Why?

Because the constant release of liver fat packages is what leads to heart attacks and strokes. Sometimes the fat packages in your blood will get stuck in the walls of your blood vessels. This is perfectly normal. One of your patrolling immune cells will notice the stuck package, take action, break it down and your waste packages will pick up the pieces and take them back to your liver.

OK.

The problems begin when fat packages start getting stuck faster than your immune cells and waste packages can deal with them. Then things start to build up: as more fat packages get stuck, more immune cells arrive and you end up with a huge chunk of fat, cholesterol, waste and immune cells, called a plaque.[13] Eventually, the plaque breaks off and floats around in your blood until it clogs up one of your blood vessels. If the clog cuts off the blood to your heart, you have a heart attack. If it cuts off the blood to your brain, you have a stroke.

I see. OK. But what makes the fat packages get stuck in the first place?

Good question. Ultimately, it's their size. This is where the concept of "good" and "bad" cholesterol comes from. It turns out that only a certain type of fat package is likely to get stuck, and that's a depleted liver fat package.[14] So when people talk about bad cholesterol, they're talking about depleted liver fat packages.

OK. But a depleted liver fat package contains more than just cholesterol, right?

Actually, by the time it's depleted, it's mostly just the cholesterol that's left,[15] so referring to it as bad cholesterol kind of makes sense.

Fine. So depleted liver fat packages are the ones that get stuck because they're the smallest?

Right.

And why is it the small packages that get stuck?

Oh, just because they are more likely to find their way into a crack. It's like rolling a golf ball and a basketball down the street. The golf ball is much more likely to get stuck in a crack, right?

OK, sure. So that's why I should keep my bad cholesterol low, so that I have fewer of these packages that are likely to get stuck.

That's right, though it turns out to be a bit more complicated than that. Even this one type of fat package comes in multiple sizes and it's actually only the small ones that are likely to get stuck. So you can have a lot of depleted liver fat packages in your blood but if they're relatively large then it doesn't matter.

OK, so the total number of depleted liver fat packages isn't that important; it's really about the number of *small* depleted liver fat packages?

Right.

OK, so what's "good" cholesterol, then?

Good cholesterol is the waste packages.

Why are they good?

Because the more of them you have in your blood, the faster you can get waste back to your liver and prevent it from building up in your blood vessels.

I see. OK, let me try to summarize.

Go ahead.

My depleted liver fat packages are my "bad cholesterol" because they can get stuck in my blood vessels.

Right. But only the small ones.

Right. When they get stuck, my immune cells will notice them and break them down and my waste packages, which are my "good cholesterol," will pick up the pieces and take them back to my liver.

Right.

But if too many of my small depleted liver fat packages are getting stuck too quickly and my immune cells and waste packages can't keep up, it all builds up into a plaque, which eventually breaks off, clogs a blood vessel and gives me a heart attack or stroke.

Exactly.

OK, I'm with you. But I don't see what this has to do with the insulin resistance you were talking about before.

Well, if you want to minimize the number of small depleted liver fat packages in your blood, insulin resistance is not going to help.[16] Remember, if your insulin isn't working, your blood fat will be high.

Oh, right. That means more fat will be passing through my liver, so it will be releasing more fat packages.[17]

Right. But not only will your liver release more fat packages, it will put more fat into those packages before it releases them.

Why does that matter?

Because the size of a fat package when it's depleted depends on how much fat it starts off with: packages that start off with more fat end up smaller when they're depleted.[18]

Packages that start off with more fat end up smaller? That's weird.

Well, remember, it's mostly just the cholesterol that's left once the package is depleted.

Oh, so packages that start off with more fat also start off with less cholesterol?

Yeah, that's a good way to think about it.[19] If the liver fat packages are all the same size to start with and it's just the cholesterol that's left when they're depleted...

Then the packages that start with the most fat and the least cholesterol will end up the smallest.

Right.

OK, I think I get it. Because my insulin isn't working anymore, my fat cells will be constantly releasing fat, so I'll have high blood fat. All of that fat in my blood will pass through my liver, which will cause my liver to release more fat packages than normal and also cause those packages to start off with more fat than normal. And that's a problem because liver fat packages that start off with a lot of fat end up smaller when they're depleted, which means they'll be likely to get stuck in my blood vessels and cause a plaque to build up.

That's right. And remember inflammation is behind it all: it causes the insulin resistance, the high blood fat and the plaque build-up.

Summary II

OK. Let me try to summarize everything, from the first big meal to the heart attack.

Go for it.

OK, so if I eat processed foods, I'll digest the glucose too quickly and my pancreas will overreact and produce too much insulin.

Right.

The glucose from the meal will get used up but, because of the extra insulin, my liver and fat cells won't start releasing glucose or fat.

Right.

So my brain will think I'm low on energy and make me feel tired and hungry so I eat again.

Right.

If this happens regularly, my fat cells will keep storing fat but never releasing it.

Right.

Eventually, when my fat cells get overwhelmed by all of the fat that they are trying to store, my immune system will step in and start interfering with my insulin, first in my fat and eventually in my whole body.

Right.

Once my insulin stops working, my liver will start constantly releasing glucose but my cells won't use any of it, so I'll have high blood glucose – that's diabetes. And my fat cells will start constantly releasing fat, so I'll have high blood fat as well.

Right.

My pancreas will try to deal with the high blood glucose by releasing more and more insulin but that won't work and eventually it will burn out.

Right.

And my liver will try to deal with the high blood fat by putting it into packages. Those packages will have a lot of fat to start off with, so they'll end up small when they get depleted and they'll be likely to get stuck in my blood vessels.

Right.

If those small depleted liver fat packages start getting stuck too fast, my immune cells and waste packages won't be able to clear them out fast enough and a plaque will build up. If the plaque gets too big, it will break off and float around until it clogs one of my blood vessels and I have a heart attack or a stroke.

Very good.

This is scary stuff.

3
Calories in

Energy signals

You're right, the problems caused by inflammation and insulin resistance are scary. But avoiding them is simple: you just need to burn more calories than you eat.

Hang on, you just told me off a few minutes ago for saying the same thing!

Not exactly. I'm saying that avoiding these problems is simple, I'm not saying it's easy. In fact, it's incredibly hard – much harder than you think. Everyone knows that people gain weight because they eat more calories than they burn. But, unfortunately, just knowing that isn't very helpful. What we need to understand are the reasons that people eat more calories than they burn. *Why* do people eat too many calories? *Why* do people burn too few calories? Unfortunately, there are a number of very powerful environmental factors and systems in your body and brain that make things very difficult.

But why? I mean, I can see how our environment with processed foods everywhere isn't helping but why would there be systems in my body and brain that want me to be unhealthy?

Well, they don't want you to be unhealthy. In fact, until very recently, they would have played an important part in keeping you healthy.

I'm confused.

That's OK, we'll go through it all step by step. The root of the problem is the environmental mismatch that I brought up earlier: the environment that our ancestors evolved in is very different from the environment we live in today. Our animal and human ancestors had to actively search for scarce, unprocessed foods, while we are surrounded by processed foods with no fiber and added sugar. Many of the systems that we're going to discuss were essential for our ancestors' survival but, in our modern environment, they've become a liability. Like the insulin overshoot that we already discussed – it simply wasn't a problem until recently. If it was, evolution would have gotten rid of it.

Right. But our environment is changing very quickly and evolution is too slow to keep up, right?

Exactly. It's really only very recently that processed foods have become such a dominant part of our diet. Maybe thousands of years from now, humans will have evolved to avoid these problems. But, right now, we're stuck with the bodies and brains we've got.

OK, let's keep going.

Good. Now, we've talked a lot about the metabolic systems that manage the energy that's in your body, but we haven't really talked about the weight regulation systems that control how much energy you take in or burn up.

You mean the systems that control how much I eat and how active I am by making me feel hungry or tired?

Exactly. There are very elaborate systems for communication between your body and brain. We'll go through the details of how these systems work and what happens when they don't. Ultimately, it always comes back to the same problem: the environmental mismatch causes us to overeat and gain weight and eventually inflammation kicks in and makes everything worse.

More inflammation?

Yup. I think the best place to start is with the systems that control when and how much you eat. First of all, there are cells in your brain that control your hunger.

OK. What part of my brain are my hunger cells in?

They're right in the middle, in an area called the hypothalamus.

Hypothalamus, got it.

The hypothalamus is really important: it has lots of different cells that control all of your bodily functions. Your hunger cells control your hunger based on signals that they receive from all over your body telling them how much energy you have.

What kind of signals?

There are a few different kinds. One set of signals comes from your stomach and intestines to tell your hunger cells about what you've eaten recently. There are nerves all over your gut that go to your brain,[1] and hormones released by your stomach and intestines.

Sorry, but I just want to make sure that I fully understand everything. What exactly is a nerve?

A nerve carries an electrical message from one place to another, like a telephone wire.

OK. So the nerves run directly from my gut to my brain. And I guess the hormones travel to my brain through my blood?

They can, yes. Or they can activate the nerves in your gut and send a signal to the brain that way. Either way.

OK, so how do these energy signals work?

Well, there are a lot of them and each one carries a different kind of message. For example, there are nerves that tell your brain how stretched out your stomach is.

That makes sense.

There are also hormones that keep track of what is coming into your blood.[2] One of the most important hormones is called ghrelin – that's your hunger hormone.[3] Ghrelin tells your brain that your stomach and intestines are empty.

OK, so if I haven't eaten in a while, my stomach and intestines will be empty and my ghrelin will be high, so my brain will make me feel hungry. As I eat, my stomach and intestines will fill up, I'll start digesting the food and my ghrelin will go down, so my brain will make me feel full. Then, after a while, when I've finished digesting, my stomach and intestines will be empty again and my ghrelin will go back up, so my brain will make me feel hungry again.

Exactly.

OK, that's pretty simple.

Good, then let's keep going. Now, the amount you eat should depend on how much energy you've already got stored, right?

You mean how much body fat I have?

Right. If you have a lot of stored fat, then you don't really need to eat, so you should feel full quickly.

Yes, that makes sense. But how can my brain know how much fat I have stored?

Your fat cells send hormones to your brain.[4]

Really?

I know, it's pretty cool, isn't it? Fat cells actually release a lot of different hormones but the most important one is called leptin – that's the fat hormone. That's the one that tells your brain how much fat you have stored. More leptin means more fat.

OK, so I guess leptin amplifies the signals from my gut, so that I feel full more quickly.

Exactly.[5]

OK, so I'll end up eating less if I'm overweight and I'll end up eating more if I'm not.

Right. And your brain also monitors a few other things: it monitors how much insulin is in your blood, since that's a good indicator of how much glucose you've eaten recently, and also how much glucose and fat are in your blood.

Right, because the whole point of my metabolic systems is to always make sure that there is enough glucose and fat in my blood to keep everything going.

Exactly.

OK, let me make sure I get it.

Go ahead.

I've got ghrelin and the other gut signals telling my brain how much food is in my gut and what's coming into my blood.

Right.

I've got leptin telling my brain how much fat I have stored.

Right.

And I've got my brain keeping its own record of how much insulin, glucose and fat are in my blood.

That's right. Those are the main energy signals that your brain uses to control your eating.

Well, that sounds like a fine system. What's the problem?

Well...

Pleasure

Wait, this gets back to the question I asked you earlier. If I'm overweight, why would I ever feel hungry at all? If I've got all that stored energy, I don't really need to eat, do I?

That's right. Since your liver can make glucose to fuel your brain and everything else can run on fat, you could, in theory, go for a long time without eating. But now we've come to the first big problem: the systems that control your eating are simply not designed for an environment in which you can eat whenever you want to.

Why not?

Well, like I said earlier, most of us have constant access to food but our ancestors didn't. They spent most of their time looking for food and, when they found some, they ate it. For them, starvation was a real risk but becoming obese was not. So their brains evolved to strongly motivate them to seek food and to eat it.

But I'm not an animal. Surely I have some control over the decision to eat or not, right? I mean, even if I'm a bit hungry, I can see food and decide not to eat it.

Yes, of course, you're right. You can always decide not to eat. You might be offered a snack and decline it because you think "Oh, I don't want to spoil my dinner" or "Oh, that looks good but I don't want to gain weight." But, given the number of people who are overweight and would rather not be, I think it's fair to say that this control is pretty weak.

So the problem is that my desire to be healthy is not strong enough to overcome my hard-wired urge to eat?

Sort of. I'd put it slightly differently. Eating – or really all behavior – is a battle between your brain's pleasure system and your brain's self-control system. Your pleasure system helps make sure that you satisfy your short-term needs by creating urges to seek pleasure or avoid unpleasantness. But your pleasure system can't see the big picture.

OK. So my pleasure system will always urge me to eat cake rather than vegetables?

Yeah, more or less. That's why you also have your self-control system: to help you ignore the urges from your pleasure system and do what's best for the long term.

Why didn't evolution just make the self-control system really strong?

That's a good question. We might get there eventually but, as you said before, evolution is really slow. Giving your self-control system all of the responsibility would require you to understand exactly what all of your needs are and organize your behavior to satisfy them, which is asking a lot. But it might work for eating.

Yeah, I think I could manage to eat enough food each day even if I didn't get much pleasure from the taste.

You might. But we inherited our brains from much simpler animals that couldn't see the big picture the way we can. So it made perfect sense for their brains to use the pleasure system to provide extra motivation to seek food and eat it because, again, starvation was a risk but obesity was not.

OK, I see what you're saying.

Good. Now, let me tell you a bit more about how your pleasure and self-control systems work.

OK.

Let's start with the pleasure system.[6] It's located deep in the middle of your brain, in the area surrounding your hypothalamus.

Does that part of the brain have a name?

Well, the pleasure system has a lot of different interconnected parts, each with its own complicated name. The names don't matter, so I think we should just keep calling it the pleasure system.

Fine.

Now, I think the first thing we need to do to understand the pleasure system is to make a distinction between "being hungry" and "wanting to eat."

What do you mean?

Well, when we talk about hunger, we're usually talking about the sensation that builds gradually after we haven't eaten for a while and that isn't necessarily linked to a specific food.

Right.

But sometimes we want to eat even when we're not hungry – maybe because we see or smell a particular food.

Oh, I see. OK, sure.

Or, even if you feel full because you just finished a meal, you might still want to eat dessert. That's different from being hungry.

Got it.

It's entirely possible, of course, to be hungry and to want to eat – in fact, that's what happens most of the time. But it's helpful to think about them separately.

OK.

So being hungry is what we've already discussed. If you haven't eaten in a while and your stomach is empty, and your ghrelin is high or your blood insulin, glucose or fat have dropped below normal levels, the hunger cells in your hypothalamus will notice and they will make you feel hungry. Alternatively, if you see something that you know is tasty, your pleasure system will make you want to eat it, whether you are hungry or not.

Hold on. It still seems like just being hungry would be enough, even for animals. Is the whole "wanting to eat" thing really necessary? I understand what you said about our brains evolving to make sure we eat enough, but they must have evolved to make sure we sleep enough as well...

That's right, I see where you're going. Just being tired at the end of each day is sufficient to get us to sleep. It's not like we get the urge to sleep every time we see a bed.

Right. So if just being tired is a strong enough signal to get us to sleep, why isn't just being hungry a strong enough signal to get us to eat?

I'm sure it would be, nowadays. The key difference is that food used to be scarce and we needed to be motivated to seek it. But that's not really the case with sleep, right?

OK, I guess we've always been more or less in control of how much we slept. We were never going to die of sleep deprivation.

Right. But if our ancestors didn't constantly put in the effort to seek food, they could easily have died of starvation. If we had evolved with constant access to food, maybe eating would be like sleeping. Maybe every morning when we woke up, we'd have a really strong urge to eat enough food for the day but we wouldn't really have any desire to eat at other times.

OK. So wanting to eat gave us the extra motivation to seek food when food was scarce, but it's not really necessary anymore.

Right. But the pleasure associated with eating isn't just about extra motivation, it's also about eating the right foods. Your human brain is capable of deciding whether something is food or not but the animals that we evolved from couldn't do that. They needed to know that eating fruit was a good idea but eating a rock was not.

OK, so if something tastes good, that's a signal that it's probably OK to eat.

Right. Now, let's get into the details of how your pleasure system works.

OK.

In order to make you want to do the things that are critical for survival – eating, sleeping, having sex, urinating and so on – your brain evolved so that doing those things is pleasant and not doing them is unpleasant. As we already discussed for eating and sleeping, the details of the pleasantness and unpleasantness might vary for the different activities but the basic idea is similar.

OK.

So wanting to eat, as opposed to being hungry, is wanting the pleasure that comes from eating. In a sense, it's no different from wanting any other form of pleasure: your brain is hard-wired to want pleasure so, if you're given the opportunity to eat something tasty, you're likely to take it. And once the urge to seek this pleasure has been triggered, it can be very hard to resist.

You almost sound like you're talking about drug addiction . . .

Ah, well, there are in fact a lot of similarities in the way food and drugs can hijack your pleasure system. We'll get into that later,

but let's talk about how your pleasure system normally controls eating first.

OK.

So your brain evolved so that eating certain foods gives you pleasure, particularly those that contain a lot of glucose or fat. Now, the link between taste and pleasure is not something your brain needs to learn: it's already there when you're born. Your taste buds are connected to nerves that send signals to your brain. When your sweet taste buds are activated, for example, they send a signal up those nerves that causes cells in your brain to release opioids and cannabinoids, which are the two pleasure chemicals.[7]

Wait, aren't those the same chemicals that are in drugs?

Yup. Opioids are in heroin and cannabinoids are in marijuana.

So my brain makes its own drugs and releases them when I eat something sweet?

Right.

OK, yeah, I can see where this is going.

Well, hold on, the fact that eating is pleasurable doesn't *need* to be a huge problem. There are plenty of pleasurable things that we can enjoy without any problems at all.

OK, sorry, go on.

So eating certain foods gives you pleasure because they taste good and that pleasure motivates you to seek and eat these foods rather than just eating other random things. What your brain needs to learn is which foods these are. It learns this pretty easily through trial and error: you try many different foods throughout your childhood and your brain remembers which taste good and which don't.

Fine.

Now, your brain is hard-wired to motivate you to seek pleasure, that's one of its most basic and powerful functions.

You really make us sound like animals!

Well, there is a really big and important part of your brain that is essentially the same as in an animal. It makes you do what you need to do to survive without having to think about it. If I described the system that allows you to breathe automatically, you wouldn't get

upset, would you? Eating is more complicated because you have to figure out how to get food but, once you've got the food, the hard-wired system can take over to make sure you eat it. Haven't you ever found yourself mindlessly munching on snacks?

OK, OK, go on.

OK. So once your brain has learned that a particular food tastes good, seeing it will trigger a craving for it.

What exactly is a craving? I mean, I know a craving is a strong desire to have something but what's actually going on in our brains?

Yes, good question; this is the key to the pleasure system. When you see something that you've learned is a source of pleasure, cells in your pleasure system release dopamine, which is the craving chemical.[8] The dopamine tells other parts of your brain, like the parts that control your movements, to do whatever they need to do to get that source of pleasure.[9]

OK.

So when you see something that you know is a source of pleasure, like tasty food, dopamine is released and triggers a craving for it. Now, because your brain is very clever, it will learn which things in your environment are typically associated with tasty food. So your pleasure system will release dopamine not only when you see the food itself but also when you see, hear or smell anything that reminds you of it.

I see; so if I walk past the kitchen and smell cookies, that might trigger a craving to go into the kitchen and eat them.

That's right. But the cues can be much more indirect than that. For example, I always have to eat Swedish Fish at the movies. I never really think about them otherwise but as soon as I enter a theater to see a movie, I crave them.

OK, that's a bit weird, but I get the point.

Good. Now, for most people, one of the most powerful food cues is the time of day. Your brain always knows more or less what time it is and if it learns that you usually eat lunch at noon, then it will make you want to eat each day around noon.

But when it's lunch time, it's not that I just want to eat, I'm usually actually hungry.

That's right. Most of your eating is partly out of hunger and partly out of just wanting to eat. Come lunch time, you might actually be hungry but you'll often want to eat something pretty specific.

Right.

And if you're pretty regular about when you eat lunch, you'll usually get hungry at the same time whether you had a big or a small breakfast.

OK, I can see how my normal lunch time might trigger a craving for food even if I had a big breakfast, but how can it actually make me hungry? If there's still food in my gut, my ghrelin should still be low and all that, right?

Right, but because your brain has learned that you usually eat at noon, it will tell your body to start preparing to digest your lunch before you even eat it.

Oh, like Pavlov's dogs started to salivate when they heard the bell, right? But, what's the point?

Right. Well, remember, your metabolic systems are all about keeping a relatively constant supply of energy in your blood. Eating, of course, is going to cause a massive increase in the amount of glucose and fat in your blood. But if your brain knows the food is coming, it can give you a head start on processing all of that glucose and fat by, for example, telling your pancreas to release insulin even before you start eating.

Oh, I see the problem. The insulin will tell my muscles to take glucose out of my blood. But because I haven't yet eaten, my blood glucose will actually drop below normal and the hunger cells in my brain will sense that and make me feel hungry.

Exactly. It's similar to the hunger that follows the insulin overshoot that we discussed earlier. And the same thing can happen with any food cue. If it happens because it's lunch time, it's not such a problem, because you're probably planning to eat anyway. But if you're watching TV in the middle of the afternoon and you see a commercial that triggers a craving *and* hunger, you're pretty likely to find yourself heading to the kitchen.

OK, I'm with you. Let me try to summarize what you've told me so far about the systems that control my hunger. I've got the energy signals that are monitored by my brain: ghrelin, leptin, insulin and blood glucose and fat.

Right.

And I've got dopamine from my pleasure system, which makes me want to eat when I see tasty food or anything that reminds me of tasty food.

Right.

And if my brain thinks that I might eat soon, it will tell my pancreas to release insulin to prepare for digestion, which, in turn, will cause my blood glucose to drop. So, I won't just want to eat, I'll also feel hungry.

Exactly.

OK. And it made sense for eating to be controlled by these signals when food was scarce because we had to be motivated to seek food and learn how to find it. But, nowadays, when food and food cues are everywhere, it's getting us into trouble.

Right. Now, there's one more thing I forgot to tell you. I told you that leptin from your fat cells amplifies the signals from your gut so that you'll feel full more quickly if you've got a lot of stored energy.

Right.

Leptin also dampens the cravings for food from your pleasure system by interfering with your dopamine.[10]

Oh, so if I'm overweight, a food cue will trigger a weaker craving, so I'll be more likely to be able to resist it?

Right. Well, at least if you're only a bit overweight. If you're really overweight and inflammation has kicked in, the whole system will break down. But we'll get to that later.

OK.

Good. Now we can move on to the self-control system.

Self-control

Your self-control system is in a different part of your brain. It's in the front of your cortex, that's the really large part of your brain behind your forehead.

Not large enough, apparently.

Well, again, the problem is the environmental mismatch. The balance between our pleasure system and our self-control system was

set based on the environment of our ancestors. Their environment had relatively few opportunities for short-term pleasure. There weren't tasty foods everywhere back then, so our ancestors' self-control systems didn't need to be that strong.

So why did the self-control system evolve in the first place?

Back then, even for animals, there was still a big advantage to behaving in a way that considered both short-term and long-term needs, rather than just responding to whatever need was most urgent at any given time. If a hungry animal found some food late in the day when it was about to get dark outside, it was more likely to survive if it could resist the urge to eat right away and take the food back to its shelter and eat it there.

I see.

That's really one of the most important functions of your self-control system: inhibiting the behaviors that are triggered by the cravings from your pleasure system in order to help you do what's best for the long term.

OK, so how does it work?

Your self-control system basically cancels the orders that are sent by your pleasure system.

How? Does it interfere with dopamine?

Not directly. What it really does is shut down the brain cells that would have carried out the order sent by the dopamine, like the cells that control your movements.[11]

OK, so it inhibits the behavior but not the craving?

Right, that's the problem: if the craving persists, your self-control will eventually break down.

Why? If I'm able to resist the craving in the first place, what changes?

Well, your brain evolved so that there would be a balance between your pleasure system and your self-control system, with each one getting its way part of the time. So if your self-control system is constantly cancelling orders, its signals will become weaker so that your pleasure system can get its way for a while. For our ancestors, this provided a good balance between short-term and long-term benefits.[12]

OK, I see. So this balance made sense for our ancestors because their pleasure systems weren't constantly getting triggered, but it's a problem for us because now there is food everywhere.

Exactly.

OK, let me try to summarize it all.

Go ahead.

Actually, wait, you told me that leptin interacts with the signals from my gut and my pleasure system so that I'll eat less if I'm overweight. Does it interact with my self-control system as well?

Oh, yes, that's right, it does. Leptin increases the strength of your self-control system so that it's more likely to be able to cancel the orders sent by your pleasure system.[13]

Summary III

Got it. OK, so let me try to go through the systems that control my eating.

Go for it.

I've got nerves and hormones from my stomach and intestines, like the hunger hormone ghrelin, that tell my brain how much I've eaten recently.

Right.

I've got the hormone leptin from my fat cells that tells my brain how much fat I have stored.

Right.

I've got insulin telling my brain how much glucose I've eaten recently.

Right.

And I've got my brain monitoring my blood glucose and fat directly to make sure they don't get too low.

Right. Those are the main energy signals.

OK. Then I've also got my pleasure system, which makes me want to eat when I see tasty food or anything that reminds me of it.

Right.

And, finally, I've got my self-control system, which can cancel the orders sent by my pleasure system.

Perfect. Now, why don't you try to run through a typical day? You've just woken up in the morning...

OK, my stomach and intestines are empty and my ghrelin is high, so the hunger cells in my hypothalamus make me feel hungry and I eat breakfast. As I eat my breakfast, my ghrelin goes down and some of the other signals from my gut go up, so I start to feel full. And, if I'm overweight, I'll feel full more quickly because my leptin will be high and it will amplify the signals from my gut.

Good, keep going. Let's say you don't have any snacks in the morning.

OK, then after a few hours when I've digested my food, my stomach and intestines will empty out, so my ghrelin will go back up and my brain will gradually start to make me feel hungry again. When my normal lunch time rolls around, I'll get really hungry because my brain has learned that I usually eat at that time, so it will start preparing for digestion. It will tell my pancreas to start releasing insulin, which will cause my muscles to start using glucose. But I haven't yet eaten anything, so my hunger cells will notice the drop in blood glucose and make me feel hungry.

Good. So you eat lunch, your gut signals do their thing again and you feel full for a while. But then in the middle of the afternoon, there's a birthday cake for someone in your office.

Right. When I see the cake, my dopamine goes up because my brain has learned that eating cake is pleasurable and my brain is hard-wired to seek pleasure. The dopamine tells the parts of my brain that control my behavior to do what is needed to eat the cake.

Good. But let's say you're worried about the fact that you've put on weight over the past couple of months.

Right. So my self-control system tries to cancel the order from my pleasure system. And since I've gained weight, my leptin is high, so it interferes with the signals from my pleasure system and boosts the strength of my self-control system and I resist the cake!

That would be good. But let's say it's your favorite kind of cake and you're unable to resist. Let's say you have a big piece of cake.

OK, well if I have a big piece of cake with a lot of easily digested glucose, I might have an insulin overshoot and, because of the extra insulin, my blood glucose and fat might end up too low. If my brain thinks that I'm low on energy, it will make me feel hungry again and maybe I'll hit the vending machine.

Right. So now it's late afternoon. You've already had breakfast, lunch, a piece of cake and now another little snack. You're full now but you're meeting a friend for dinner...

Right. And when I get to the restaurant, my brain knows that restaurants mean food so it starts preparing for digestion again. My insulin goes up, my blood glucose goes down and, even though I'm still pretty full, I start feeling hungry, so I eat.

Right. I mean, you're at a restaurant – of course you're going to eat, right? OK, then finally, after dinner, you see some really good-looking desserts being taken to the next table.

No, no way. This time I'm not giving in. My stomach and intestines are full. My pleasure system has had its way all day long. This time my self-control system is cancelling the order sent by my pleasure system.

OK, fair enough. Great job with the summary.

Thanks, I think I'm starting to get it now. I can really see why it's so hard to eat right.

Well, so far we've only discussed how eating is controlled when things are working well. It can get much, much harder. I mentioned the similarities between food and drugs before, so let's go back to that.

OK.

Addiction

So we've talked about how your pleasure system can trigger cravings far too often because our modern environment has food or reminders of food everywhere.

Right.

But, even still, most of us would probably be fine if food didn't taste so good.

What do you mean?

Well, the strength of the craving triggered by a particular food depends on the pleasure associated with eating it. If our environment was full of bland foods, our pleasure system wouldn't trigger so many cravings because eating bland food is not that pleasurable.

OK.

But our pleasure system is calibrated for the kinds of foods that our ancestors would have eaten. These foods were typically pretty bland compared to the processed foods we eat today, which have a lot of added sugar. The problem is that sugar just tastes too good. It's off the charts. The pleasure we get from eating processed foods with added sugar is totally unnatural.

I see.

And it's simply too much for some people. For them, food can hijack the pleasure system, just like a drug can.[14]

So are you going to tell me that some people get addicted to food? That sounds a bit far-fetched.

Does it? There are a lot of obese people who show all of the signs of addiction. They're fully aware that they shouldn't be eating so much and they would love to stop but they can't – they just keep doing it. And if they're prevented from eating, they'll have strong cravings and it will be extremely unpleasant.

C'mon. Sugar is not cocaine.

No, it's not. But the point is that they both give rise to an unnaturally strong feeling of pleasure and, because of that, they can cause unnaturally strong cravings. Drugs might be more powerful than sugar or other tasty foods but sugar has the "advantage" that it's connected with eating, which is something that your brain is hardwired to make you want to do.

OK. But I thought that one of the key things with drug addiction was that you build up a tolerance, so that you have to keep taking more and more of the drug just to get the same high.

That's right; if you take a lot of drugs, your pleasure chemicals – the opioids or the cannabinoids – will be high all of the time, so your brain will stop paying attention to them. As you said, this means that the drug becomes less effective, so you need to keep taking more and more of it to get the same high.

Right.

But it's only your pleasure chemicals that your brain stops paying attention to, not your dopamine. So even though the drug is less effective, you still have the same strong craving for it.

Right. So some addicts get to a point where they'll desperately seek whatever it is that they're addicted to but then they won't even enjoy it when they get it. And you're telling me that the same thing happens with food?

Yes, for some people. As you become obese, it's likely that your brain will start releasing more dopamine when you see food and fewer opioids and cannabinoids when you actually eat it.[15] So you'll constantly be craving food but you won't actually enjoy it that much when you eat it.

So are all obese people addicted to food?

No, no, definitely not. But addiction is not an all or nothing thing. There isn't anything about an addicted brain that is clearly different from a normal brain. There's no blood test or brain scan for addictions – they're diagnosed based on behavior. Basically, if your behavior suggests that your pleasure system has become totally dominant over your self-control system, you'll be diagnosed with an addiction. But even if your behavior doesn't officially qualify you as addicted, it can still be a real problem.

Sure. So why is it that some people get addicted to food and others don't?

Well, part of it is genetic. Some people have relatively strong pleasure systems or relatively weak self-control systems.[16] But the real problem is our modern environment. If there was no such thing as processed foods with added sugar, hardly anyone would have a problem. But because unnaturally tasty food is literally everywhere, we're all at risk.

Right.

And there are also other environmental factors that are not directly related to food that can tip the balance in favor of the pleasure system.

Like what?

Stress

Like stress.

Oh, yeah. I know a lot of people who eat when they're stressed.

Exactly. "Comfort foods" got their name for a good reason.[17]

So eating actually does relieve stress?

It definitely can, at least for a little while. Maybe I should explain a bit about how the stress system works.[18]

Yes, please do.

Whenever you sense a threat, your brain responds by releasing chemicals that are meant to help you cope with that threat.

Like adrenaline?

Exactly.

Adrenaline gives me extra strength, right? So I can run away from a lion or lift up a car before my baby is crushed.

Yeah, sort of. Adrenaline helps get extra energy to your muscles by telling your liver to make and release glucose and your fat cells to release fat. In that sense, it's sort of an anti-insulin. Adrenaline also does a lot of other things and it's obviously important but, when it comes to the effects of stress on eating, there is another chemical that is much more important: cortisol.

Oh, OK. What does cortisol do?

Cortisol does a lot of different things. Most importantly, it makes you act on instinct.

Because if I'm being chased by a lion, I don't want to think, I just want to run.

Exactly. And acting on instinct is really useful if you are, in fact, facing a physical threat. But that kind of stress is relatively rare these days. Most of our stress is mental stress. In fact, there are a lot of people who are under mental stress pretty much constantly.

Yeah, I might know someone like that...

Right. If you are constantly under stress and your cortisol is constantly high, that means that you're constantly going to be acting on

instinct. Now, what do you think "acting on instinct" means in terms of eating?

I guess it means letting my pleasure system control my eating?

Exactly. Cortisol tips the balance between your pleasure and self-control systems in favor of your pleasure system.[19]

OK, so if I'm stressed and my cortisol is high, I'm much more likely to give in to my cravings for tasty food.

Right.

OK, that's not good.

No, it's not.

So how does cortisol work? Does it boost my pleasure system? Or does it interfere with my self-control system?

Both, actually. Cortisol boosts the amount of dopamine released by your pleasure system and it blocks the ability of your self-control system to cancel the orders sent by your pleasure system.[20]

Double trouble.

Exactly. And the consequences can be pretty severe, and often perverse – like for people who stress about their weight.

What do you mean?

A lot of people are constantly worried about their weight, even people who aren't overweight, and rightfully so. We've discussed how risky the modern environment is. If you're not constantly on your guard, it's easy to become overweight and unhealthy.

Right, so in order to avoid eating the tasty foods that are everywhere, I have to constantly use my self-control system to cancel the orders sent by my pleasure system.

Right, and that's really hard to do, so constantly trying to resist your cravings and worrying about the consequences every time you give in to them can easily become a source of stress. But, in this case, the stress response can really backfire.

Right. Because if I'm stressed and my cortisol is high, it will tip the balance in favor of my pleasure system and make it even harder for me to resist my cravings.

Exactly. And, to make matters worse, eating tasty foods really does reduce your stress temporarily, so you might start to use it as a regular coping strategy.

How does eating tasty food reduce stress?

The opioids and cannabinoids released by your pleasure system will actually shut down your stress system. So any pleasurable activity would probably help to reduce stress but eating tasty foods is really effective.

I see. But why would opioids and cannabinoids shut down my stress system?

Well, the links between stress, pleasure and survival might be relatively weak for us nowadays, but that wasn't the case for our ancestors: they were stressed by actual threats to their survival and got pleasure from doing things they actually needed to do to survive ...

Oh, so if my pleasure system is releasing opioids and cannabinoids, my brain thinks that I've successfully dealt with the threat?

Right. But, of course, it's really only a short-term solution. If the threat is still there, the stress will return.

Ah, right. Until I eat something tasty again. But if I do this repeatedly, I'm going to start gaining weight. And if I start gaining weight, eating is going to become an even bigger source of stress, so I'm going to find it harder and harder to resist my cravings. It's a vicious cycle.

Exactly. And it can get even worse. If you're stressed out all the time, your brain will recognize that the cortisol isn't cutting it and it will start trying other ways to tip the balance towards your pleasure system.

Like what?

It will literally make your pleasure system bigger and your self-control system smaller.[21]

Whoa.

Yeah. And once that's done, it can be hard to undo, even if you manage to eliminate the source of the stress. So the influence of stress on the balance between your pleasure system and your self-control system can last long after the stress itself is gone.

Right, so stress is bad news. I always see stories about links between stress and heart attacks, but that's not just because of the effects of stress on eating, is it?

Oh no, there is a lot more to it. For example, if your cortisol is always high, it will cause the fat from other parts of your body to move to your belly.[22]

What? OK, first of all, why would that ever be helpful in coping with a threat? And, second of all, why would that be bad for me? Fat is fat, right?

Well, belly fat cells are slightly different from fat cells in other parts of your body[23] **because they can release their stored energy more quickly. Do you remember what we just said about adrenaline?**

It tells my liver to release glucose and my fat cells to release fat.

Right, and belly fat cells are more sensitive to adrenaline than other fat cells. So in the old days, if our ancestors were constantly under threat and often needed quick access to their stored energy, it was better to keep it stored in belly fat.

OK, I guess that makes sense. But why is belly fat more of a problem than any other fat? Oh, hold on, you've got that look on your face that you always get before you start talking about inflammation.

Do I? Yes, the problem is inflammation. Belly fat is more easily inflamed than fat in other parts of your body and the chemicals released by the immune cells in your belly fat can easily leak out into your liver.[24]

Oh, OK, hold on, let me take a shot at this. The chemicals from my immune cells can interfere with my insulin, so if my belly fat is inflamed it can cause insulin resistance in my liver.

Right.

Normally, when my insulin is low, my liver releases glucose. And the insulin resistance will make my liver think that my insulin is low, even when it's actually high. So that means if I have insulin resistance in my liver, it will release glucose constantly.

Right, so you'll end up with high blood glucose. And don't forget, your belly fat is inflamed as well.

Right, and my inflamed belly fat will be constantly releasing fat, which will also go straight into my liver?

Right.

Oh, right, I see the link to heart attacks now. My liver will put the fat that's coming from my belly into the packages that it makes. So my liver fat packages will start off with a lot of fat, which means they'll end up smaller when they're depleted and they'll be more likely to get stuck in my blood vessels, lead to a build-up of plaque and, eventually, a heart attack or stroke.

Exactly.

OK, I get the picture.

Leptin resistance

Good. That's enough about stress for now; we'll come back to it again when we talk about exercise. But since you brought up inflammation again...

What?

OK, since we've started discussing inflammation again, I think this is a good time to discuss the consequences of brain inflammation.[25]

Oh, my brain can get inflamed too?

Sure. Your brain has its own private immune system but it's more or less the same as your body's immune system. Do you remember what we said about inflammation in the body?

I think so. If I overeat, my cells will get overwhelmed with glucose and fat and they won't be able to process it fast enough. So if I keep overeating, I'll get a build-up of waste and half-processed glucose and fat. My immune cells will take notice and they'll interfere with my insulin to prevent my muscle cells from taking in more glucose and my fat cells from trying to store more fat, giving them a chance to clear out the backlog. It's OK if this happens once in a while but, if it's happening all the time, then my insulin won't ever work properly and I'll have all kinds of problems.

Good. Now, the same thing happens in your brain with overeating leading to inflammation and insulin resistance. But when your immune cells interfere with the insulin in your brain, it causes a different set of problems.

Like what?

Well, most importantly, when your immune cells interfere with the insulin in your brain, they also interfere with leptin. So you won't just have insulin resistance, you'll also have leptin resistance.[26]

Why?

Because your brain cells use the same escort for insulin and leptin,[27] so it's impossible to interfere with one without also interfering with the other.

Ugh.

And you remember what leptin does, right?

Yeah, I remember. It tells my brain how much fat I have stored. I'll eat less if my leptin is high because it will boost the signals from my gut so that I feel full more quickly. And it will also interfere with the dopamine from my pleasure system and strengthen my self-control system so that my cravings will be weaker and I'll be more able to resist them.

Right. So do you see where this is going?

Yup. My leptin will fail me right when I need it the most. If I'm overeating consistently and my brain becomes inflamed, the one signal that would have helped me eat less disappears.

Actually, it's even worse than that. If your leptin isn't working, your brain will think that you are low on stored energy, so it will actually push you to eat more.

Oh, wow. OK, you're not going to try to argue that this makes some kind of evolutionary sense, are you?

No, not really. It's very common for cells to use the same escort for different things, it's just unfortunate that leptin and insulin happen to use the same one. But remember, this problem never would have arisen for our ancestors. They never would have had the constant inflammation that we do because they never would have consistently overeaten the way that we do.

Right.

4
Calories out

Weight regulation

Now, when inflammation causes leptin resistance, it doesn't only affect your brain's ability to control how much you eat, it also affects your brain's ability to control how much energy you burn.

OK. We haven't really talked about how my brain controls how much energy I burn.

Right, I think it's time we do. The important thing to keep in mind is that when things are working properly, your weight regulation systems try to match how many calories you eat and how many calories you burn.

Really?

What do you mean, "really?" We've talked about the different systems that control your eating. We just finished talking about leptin a second ago.

I know. And I understand how leptin will help me eat less if I start gaining weight. But doesn't the fact that most people are overweight suggest that these systems don't really do all that much?

No! It's true that most people are overweight but there are still a lot of people who aren't. And even those that do gain weight still typically gain only a few pounds per year. Do you realize how remarkable that is? Even if you gain a few pounds per year, the number of calories that you eat and the number that you burn are still incredibly closely matched.

Well...

Hold on. To gain a pound per year, you need to eat 3500 more calories than you burn.[1] If you spread that out over the whole year it comes out to about 10 calories per day. That's nothing! That's not even a tiny bite of food.

So what are you saying?

I'm saying that most people have no clue about the number of calories they're eating and burning each day, yet they are able to match these numbers to within a bite of food. Do you think that is just a coincidence?

I guess not.

It's not a coincidence at all. It's because our weight regulation systems are incredibly effective at matching the number of calories that we eat and the number that we burn, even when we make their job extremely difficult by living in an environment that's very different from the one they were designed for. These systems only break down after we've pushed things way too far and inflammation has kicked in.

OK, calm down.

Sorry. It's just completely unreasonable to blame our problems on our weight regulation systems. We should really be blaming ourselves for creating an environment that has caused these systems to fail. If you were sitting inside a freezer and felt cold, would you blame your body's temperature control systems for failing to keep you warm?

OK, OK, I see what you're saying.

Anyway, let's get back on track. So your weight regulation systems try to match the number of calories that you eat and burn to keep your weight constant. Now, it's true that these systems are much more tolerant of weight gain than they are of weight loss – I'm not trying to argue otherwise. But I hope you're convinced by now that that this made sense in the environment we evolved in.

Sure.

Good. But it's also kind of an obvious point. There's just a lot more room for weight gain than there is for weight loss. A lean person who gains 50 or even 100 pounds can survive for years but a lean person cannot lose 50 or 100 pounds; it's just not possible.

Right. But how do my weight regulation systems choose what weight they try to maintain?

That's a good question. It's largely genetic: different people will have different natural weights.[2] Maybe you're lucky and you can maintain a six-pack without even thinking about it. Or maybe you're unlucky and you're doomed to be a bit soft around the middle no matter what you do.

But most people's natural weight is in the healthy range, right?

Oh, sure. If you're overweight, it's not because your natural weight is too high. It's because the systems that try to maintain your natural weight have broken down. For example, leptin tells your brain how much fat you have stored, so it's one of the key signals that your brain uses to determine where you stand relative to your natural weight. But if your brain thinks your leptin is low because your immune cells are interfering with it, then it will think that you are below your natural weight even if you're not, and the systems that control how many calories you eat and how many you burn will act to make you gain weight when you should be losing it.

Got it.

Good. Before we discuss the different systems that control how many calories you burn, I think we need to discuss the different ways that you use energy.

Wait, hold on, let me ask a question first. What exactly is a calorie?

Oh, it's just a measure of energy, like a mile is a measure of distance.

Oh, OK, sorry. Please go on.

OK. So most of the energy you burn is spent just keeping your body going.

Like keeping my heart beating and all that?

Right. Even people who exercise a lot still burn most of their calories just staying alive.

OK.

Good. Now, the amount of energy that you need to stay alive will depend on how much of your body is muscle and how much is fat.

Why does that matter?

Because muscle cells burn more calories just staying alive than fat cells do.

So putting on muscle can help me lose weight.

Well, putting on muscle is never a bad idea. But it won't necessarily help you lose weight. If you need more calories, you brain will just make you hungrier, right? If you put on muscle and start burning more calories without also eating more, you'll start burning your stored fat…

But then my leptin will drop and I'll start eating more to compensate until I get back to my natural weight.

Right. And not only would you start eating more when your leptin dropped, you'd also start using less energy.

How?

Fidgeting

Your brain can control how much energy you use.

Sure. That's kind of obvious, right? I have to decide to exercise and deciding requires a brain.

Right. And self-control of exercise is important but, just as with control of eating, a lot of the ways that your brain controls how much energy you use are automatic.

OK. So sometimes I'll just find myself taking the stairs rather than the elevator without really having thought about it?

Right. But it goes way beyond that to things that you wouldn't even notice.

Like what?

Like pacing or even fidgeting?

Fidgeting?

Yes, fidgeting. Most people burn hundreds of calories per day just fidgeting.[3]

What?

You know, shifting position, tapping your foot, whatever…

I know what fidgeting is, I just had no idea it burned so many calories.

Oh, definitely.

So, if I want to burn more calories, I should try to fidget more?

Well, if you're trying to do it, it's not really fidgeting – it's exercising. I suppose it might help if we could train ourselves to fidget more without thinking about it but that doesn't seem possible.

So what determines how much I fidget?

Well, part of it is genetic; some people just tend to fidget more than others.[4] But it also depends on whether or not your weight regulation systems think you need to be wasting energy.

And what part of my brain controls fidgeting, is it the hypothalamus again?

That's right, there are fidget cells in the hypothalamus.[5]

And let me guess: they are sensitive to leptin, right? So if I start gaining weight and my leptin goes up, the high leptin will tell my fidget cells to make me fidget more so that I burn more calories and return to my natural weight.

Exactly. And, of course, if you keep overeating and your brain gets inflamed, your leptin will stop working and this system will fail.

Right.

Wasting energy

Good. Now, we can get to the really interesting part. Your brain doesn't just control how active you are, it also controls how much energy you actually use during a given activity.

You mean like how fast I run or walk?

No, that's not what I mean. Even if you are running or walking at a constant speed, your brain can tell your cells to use more or less energy.[6]

I don't understand.

Well, when your cells use glucose or fat for energy, only part of the energy is actually used to make you move – the rest is used to create heat.

Why?

To keep you warm.

Oh, sure, I guess that's the point of shivering when you're really cold.

Exactly. And, as you might imagine, the amount of energy that is used to create heat depends on how cold it is outside.

That makes sense.

So that means that the same amount of movement can burn a different number of calories. For example, if you burn 500 calories running a few miles in warm weather, you might burn 600 calories running the same distance at the same speed in cold weather, because you used an extra 100 calories keeping warm.

It can really make that big of a difference?

Oh, sure.

OK, so if it's cold, my brain will tell my cells to create a lot of heat. But, if it's warm, my brain will tell my cells not to bother.

Right.

How can my brain send a signal to all of my cells like that?

The usual ways: hormones or nerves.

Fine. So you're telling me that if I want to lose weight, I should move to the North Pole?

No. Even if you did burn more calories up there, you'd probably just eat more to make up for it. If you started losing weight, you're leptin would go down and . . .

It was just a joke.

Oh. Right. Anyway, the important point here has nothing to do with temperature. Your brain also tells your cells to create more or less heat depending on how much energy you have stored. If you start gaining weight, your brain will tell your cells to waste energy by creating heat so that you'll burn more calories and return to your natural weight. If you start losing weight, your brain will tell your cells to save energy by not creating heat, so that you'll burn fewer calories and return to your natural weight.

Really?

Yes.

Is this really that important? I mean, how many calories are we actually talking about?

Yes, it's important. We're talking about hundreds of calories per day.[7]

But...

Hold on, I want to make sure that you understand how important this is. Most of us eat *many* more calories each day than we need, so the only reason that we're able to stay lean or gain weight relatively slowly, is because our brains are constantly telling our cells to waste as much as energy as they can.

Really?

Really. But, of course, the amount of energy that our cells can waste is limited. So if we just keep eating too much and doing too little, we're going to end up overweight eventually.

Wow, OK. This whole thing is pretty amazing. I really had no idea that my brain could control how many calories my cells burn like that.

I agree, it is pretty amazing. Now, as I'm sure you've guessed, this amount of energy that your cells waste by creating heat is controlled by your hypothalamus and leptin.[8] If your leptin is high, your hypothalamus will tell your cells to waste energy. If your leptin is low, your hypothalamus will tell your cells to save energy.

OK.

So do you see the problem? This is one of the main reasons why it's so hard to lose weight once inflammation has kicked in. If your leptin stops working, your brain will think that your leptin is low and it will tell your muscles to save energy instead of wasting it.

Oh, I see. So it will be much harder for me to lose weight because it will be much harder for me to burn calories. I'll burn fewer calories doing the same amount of activity than I would if my leptin was working ...

Right. You'll burn *hundreds of calories per day* fewer than you would if your leptin was working. That's the equivalent of eating a small meal or of jogging a few miles. So if your leptin isn't working and you want to lose weight, you have to eat *a lot* less or exercise *a lot* more than you would otherwise, which is just really, really hard to do for any extended period of time.

Right.

This is why most people who lose weight just end up regaining it.[9] You might be able to burn more calories than you eat for a few weeks but if your brain thinks your leptin is low and all of the systems that control the number of calories that you eat and burn start pushing for you to regain the weight, it's going to be really hard not to.[10]

Right. OK. Let me try to summarize.

Summary IV

Go ahead.

If I overeat consistently, my brain will get inflamed and my leptin won't work anymore.

Right.

So my brain will think my leptin is low even though it's actually high.

Right.

Which means my brain will think that I'm below my natural weight, even though I'm actually above it.

Right.

So the systems that control how much I eat and how much energy I burn will act to make me gain weight.

Right.

I'll eat more than I should because it'll take more food for my gut signals to make me feel full. And the cravings from my pleasure system will be strong while the ability of my self-control system to resist them will be weak.

Right.

I'll also burn fewer calories because I'll be less active and I'll fidget less.

Right.

And whatever activity I do will burn fewer calories than it should because my brain will tell my cells to save energy when they should be wasting it.

Right.

And these effects add up to hundreds of calories per day. So if I want to lose weight but my brain is inflamed and my leptin isn't working, I'll have to eat a lot less or work out a lot more than I would otherwise.

Excellent. I hope you're starting to see the big picture now.

Yeah, I think I am. First of all, staying lean is really difficult because our modern environment is very different from the one we evolved in. Instead of being forced to actively search for scarce, unprocessed foods like our ancestors, we're surrounded by processed foods.

Right. And why exactly are processed foods a problem?

Well, first of all, processed foods have usually had their fiber removed, which means they're too easy to digest. When I eat them, my blood glucose jumps and my pancreas overreacts and releases too much insulin. Because of the extra insulin, my blood glucose actually ends up below normal and my fat cells are prevented from releasing fat, so my brain thinks that I'm low on energy and makes me feel hungry and tired so that I eat more calories and burn fewer.

Good. Is that it?

No, the other big problem is that processed foods have a lot of added sugar. A lot of added sugar means a lot of fructose, which gets turned straight to fat in my liver, where it builds up and gets put into liver fat packages. And this is a problem because liver fat packages that start with a lot of fat end up smaller and more likely to get stuck in my blood vessels when they're depleted. The added sugar also makes processed foods tastier than unprocessed foods, so they activate my pleasure system really strongly and are harder for me to resist.

Good.

OK. But even though staying lean is difficult, it's nothing compared to trying to lose weight once inflammation has kicked in. Once inflammation is preventing my insulin and leptin from working, all of the systems that should be helping me to lose weight by eating less and burning more calories actually start pushing me to eat more and burn fewer calories.

Exactly!

Exercise

It sounds pretty hopeless.

Oh, no, it's not hopeless at all. Very difficult for sure but not hopeless. We haven't yet talked about our most powerful tool for weight regulation: exercise!

Right but I don't see how exercise can be all that helpful. If I exercise a lot and start burning more calories, I'm just going to eat more to make up the difference, right?

Only if you are below your natural weight. If you are above your natural weight and your insulin and leptin are still working properly, then your brain is going to let you burn the extra calories to get back to your natural weight. In fact, your brain is going to push you to exercise.[11]

What part of my brain controls how much I exercise? Is it the hypothalamus again?

Not really. The hypothalamus controls how many calories you burn automatically in the ways that we already discussed. When you choose to exercise, that's a decision that's controlled by the balance between your pleasure system and your self-control system, just like with eating.

Oh, OK – hold on then. If exercise is such a good thing, why didn't evolution make it pleasurable?

It did! If your weight regulation systems are actually working properly, then exercise is pleasurable.[12]

Oh, c'mon …

I'm serious. When things are working properly, exercise will cause your brain to release opioids and cannabinoids, just the way that eating tasty food would. Haven't you heard of "runner's high?"[13]

Sure. But…

Well, that's a very clear example. The pleasure from exercise might not always be that intense but, if your weight regulation systems are working properly, and you have extra calories that you need to burn, you will enjoy it.

I'm sorry, I just don't believe you. There is simply no way that I could ever enjoy the elliptical machine, it's just torture.

Who said anything about the elliptical machine? That is exercise, of course, and I totally agree that it's torture. But I'm not talking about that kind of exercise. I'm talking about the kind of exercise that we evolved to do.

You mean what our ancestors needed to be motivated to do in order to find food?

Exactly. Walking outdoors. Or maybe jogging, if they needed to cover a lot of ground.

OK, I guess I can believe that something like hiking could be pleasurable. Wait, so are you saying that most people don't like exercise because they are out of shape?

Sort of. But it's more than being in or out of shape. I'm saying that if your brain is inflamed, it will make exercise unpleasant because it will think that you are underweight and it won't want you to burn any extra calories.

Really?

Sure. Your brain uses your pleasure system to make sure that you do what you need to do to survive, so whether something is pleasant or unpleasant can change depending on what your brain thinks your needs are. A good example is the taste of salt water. Normally, it's disgusting but if you get really low on salt, it will start to taste just as good as something sweet.[14]

I didn't know that. OK, so this is yet another reason that I should do whatever I can to lose weight before inflammation kicks in.

Right. Because, remember, every time you use your self-control system to overrule your pleasure system it becomes harder to do it again the next time. When exercising goes from being pleasant to being unpleasant, the decision to exercise goes from being a decision that your pleasure system supports to being a decision that it opposes.

Oh, I see. So if I enjoy my exercise, I'll have an easier time using my self-control system to resist a craving for a snack later in the day. But if I have to force myself to exercise, that craving is going to be hard to resist.

Exactly.

Ugh. So what can I do if inflammation has already kicked in?

Well, first you need to recognize that everything is going to be *much* harder because your weight regulation systems are going to fight you every step of the way. Your number one priority has to be to decrease your inflammation, since that is what is causing all the problems.

And how do I do that?

Well, since your excess body fat is the source of the inflammation, losing some weight is a good place to start.

Yeah, sure. But how do I do that?

Well, of course, if you want to lose weight and decrease your inflammation, you need to burn more calories than you eat. That's going to be very difficult for all of the reasons that we've discussed. But exercise is going to help a lot, not only because it will help you burn more calories but also because it will decrease your inflammation directly.[15]

Really? Why?

Well, exercise can be very difficult for your muscles. When they're trying to use glucose and fat for energy as fast as they can, things get a bit messy. It's just like overeating: you end up with a lot of half-processed glucose and fat and a lot of waste.

So doesn't that increase inflammation rather than decrease it?

It does at first, but then your brain will send out a signal to decrease the inflammation and that decrease can be a lot stronger and last a lot longer than the initial increase, especially if you exercise hard.

I see. So how does my brain send a signal to decrease the inflammation like that?

Cortisol.

The stress hormone?

That's right. Cortisol is very good at decreasing inflammation. In fact, it's often given to people as a medicine for that purpose.

Isn't that cortisone?

Same thing.

OK, hold on. First of all, why not just give overweight people cortisol to help decrease their inflammation? And second of all, if cortisol decreases inflammation, then why isn't stress a good thing?

Well, in both cases, the problem is that the cortisol stops decreasing inflammation after a while. It's obvious with the medicine and it's also true with mental stress. It's very hard to outsmart your brain. Cortisol isn't just a stand-alone chemical; it's part of a system designed to deal with stress, which, for our ancestors, meant actual physical threats. Dealing with physical threats usually requires intense activity, like running or fighting, that causes inflammation in your muscles, and cortisol is released to decrease that inflammation.

Like with exercise?

Exactly. But if your brain notices that there is a lot of cortisol around even when there is no inflammation in your muscles from physical activity then it thinks the system has gotten out of balance and it takes measures to weaken the effect of the cortisol.[16]

But this doesn't happen with exercise?

No, because exercise causes the kind of inflammation in your muscles that cortisol is meant to decrease, so your brain is happy with the way the system is working.

Oh, I see. OK, so exercise is important because it burns calories and it decreases inflammation.

Those are the biggest benefits, but there are so many others... [17]

Like what?

Well, when you exercise regularly, your body makes a lot of changes to help get energy to your muscles more quickly.

Such as...

Such as making your blood vessels stronger so blood can travel through them more quickly. As a result, your blood vessels will have fewer cracks and your depleted liver fat packages will be less likely to get stuck.

Nice.

Yeah. And in order to help get energy from your fat cells to your muscles, your body will build new blood vessels in between your fat cells.

Oh, that's going to help decrease inflammation, right?

Yes, very good. Your immune cells take action when they notice that your fat cells are dying because they're too far from any blood vessels to get the oxygen they need. So if you build more blood vessels in between your fat cells, fewer of them are going to die and your inflammation is going to decrease. I could go on and on about the benefits of exercise but you get the point, right?

Yeah, I guess; we can move on.

5
Gut bacteria

Gut bacteria

Good. Now, we've covered almost all of the different systems that are important for metabolism and weight regulation.

Great, so what's left?

Gut bacteria!

What makes you like gut bacteria so much?

Oh, I don't know. I guess it's the fact that we still have so much to learn about them. They do _much_ more than we could have imagined even just a few years ago and it seems like we find out something new about them every week.[1]

OK, well, if you're excited then I'm excited. What exactly are bacteria anyway?

Bacteria are tiny living things. They're usually just one cell with one job: they take in one chemical and release another, stealing a little energy for themselves in the process.

OK. And we're supposed to be afraid of them, right? Isn't that why we wash with soap, because it kills bacteria?

Some bacteria are dangerous because the chemicals they release are poisonous, but most bacteria are harmless. You have to understand how many bacteria are out there.[2] They're everywhere. There are more bacteria on Earth than animals and plants combined.

But they're so small...

I don't mean by number, I mean by weight.

Oh.

And you have a huge number of bacteria on you and in you – about 100 trillion, which is 10 times the number of human cells in your body.[3] And all together they weigh a few pounds – as much as your brain.

Really?

Yup. And most of them are in your gut, particularly in your intestines.

Are they all the same kind? Do they all take in and release the same chemicals?

Oh no, there are many different kinds with many different jobs. We haven't even identified them all yet.

OK, so what do they do?

A lot of different things. But one of their most important jobs is to help with digestion. Do you remember what we said about digestion?

I think so. My mouth and my stomach break down the food I eat into a half-digested mush.

Right.

My stomach sends chunks of the mush into my intestines where the carbs are broken down into glucose and fructose and the fats are broken down into fatty acids.

Right.

The glucose and fructose go straight into my blood as is. And the fatty acids go into my blood after getting repackaged together with cholesterol.

Right.

And... oh, right, hold on, you never told me what happens to fiber.

Right, that's why I brought it up again. One thing we've known about gut bacteria for a long time is that they digest fiber.

So you mean they take in fiber and release something else?

Exactly. They take in fiber and release fat.

Fat?

That's right. And this fiber fat is really important.[4] You can digest fiber fat and use it for energy just like any other fat, but that's not really why it's important. It's important because the cells that make up the walls of your intestines don't get their energy from the glucose or fat in your blood, they get their energy directly from the fiber fat made by your gut bacteria.

I see. And presumably my gut bacteria get something out of it as well, right?

Oh, sure. They keep some energy from the fiber for themselves to survive.

So everybody wins.

Or everybody loses. If you don't eat enough fiber, your gut bacteria will die and your intestinal wall cells won't have enough energy.

Right. What happens then?

Your intestinal wall cells won't work properly if they don't have enough energy, and that can be a serious problem because they have a lot of important jobs. First of all, your intestinal wall cells decide what does and doesn't get into your blood. They need to let glucose, fat and other things from food into your blood while keeping other harmful things out. If they stop working properly, all kinds of things will get into your blood that shouldn't be there. And you know what happens then, right?

Inflammation!

Exactly. Your patrolling immune cells will detect the things that aren't supposed to be there and they'll take action. This kind of inflammation from a leaky gut is a major problem for people who don't eat a lot of fiber, which is, of course, most people.[5]

Right, because a lot of processed foods have had their fiber removed.

Right. And your intestine is a particularly bad spot to have inflammation because it's so close to your liver.

Oh, so it's like with belly fat. If my intestine is inflamed, the chemicals from my immune cells will leak into my liver and interfere with the insulin there.

Right.[6]

Fiber

OK, so that's why the fiber in unprocessed foods is important? Because it feeds the bacteria that feed my intestinal wall cells?

Well, the fiber in unprocessed foods is important for a lot of reasons.[7] In addition to feeding the bacteria that feed your intestinal wall cells, it also slows digestion, which will help your pancreas to be able to track the amount of glucose coming into your blood more accurately.

Oh, right, because it takes time to break down the fiber and release the glucose that's inside of it.

Right. And another reason that the fiber in unprocessed foods is important, especially if you're trying to lose weight, is simply that it isn't glucose, fructose or fat.

What do you mean?

Well, while you do get some calories out of fiber from the fat that your bacteria make, you get a lot fewer calories than you do from the same amount of glucose, fructose or fat. So processed foods that have had their fiber removed are much more calorie dense than unprocessed foods.

What do you mean by calorie dense?

I mean that foods without fiber have more calories per bite than foods with fiber.

Why does that matter?

Because some of the energy signals that your gut sends to your brain – for example, the nerves that tell your brain how stretched out your stomach is – only measure how much food you eat, not how many calories are in it.[8] So if you eat unprocessed foods with fiber, you'll feel full after fewer calories than if you eat processed foods with no fiber.[9]

OK, hold on, this sounds too good to be true. If I switch from processed foods to unprocessed foods and start losing weight because I'm eating fewer calories, then my weight regulation systems will just find a way to make up the difference, won't they?

Maybe, maybe not. If you're lean and those systems are working properly then, yes, you might just end up back at your natural

weight. But if your weight regulation systems aren't working properly because you're overweight and inflammation has kicked in, then eating a lot of fiber might help.

OK, I guess I can see that.

But even if you're only a bit overweight, eating a lot of fiber can still help.

How?

Well, if you want to lose weight then you need to burn the extra fat that is stored in your fat cells, right?

Right.

But your fat cells only release fat when your insulin is low, right?

Right.

So eating less glucose will help because your pancreas will release less insulin, right?

Right.

Good. Now, if you're trying to burn the fat that is stored in your fat cells, you don't really want to replace glucose with fat because that would sort of defeat the purpose and you don't want to replace glucose with fructose because that will cause other problems. But if you replace glucose with fiber, that might help a lot.

I see. So I'm better off eating unprocessed foods with fiber and glucose instead of processed foods with just glucose not only because I might end up eating fewer calories overall but also because I'll end up eating less glucose overall, which means my pancreas will release less insulin overall and my fat cells will start releasing fat again sooner than they would otherwise.

Exactly.

OK, let me see if I get it. Eating unprocessed foods with fiber instead of processed foods with no fiber is good for a lot of reasons. First of all, the fiber will feed my gut bacteria and keep my intestinal wall cells healthy, which will prevent my gut from becoming leaky and inflamed.

Right.

Second of all, the fiber in unprocessed foods also makes them less calorie dense than processed foods. So, since some of my energy signals only measure how much food I eat rather than how many calories are in it, I'm likely to feel full after eating fewer calories.

Right.

And, finally, eating unprocessed foods with fiber will also help keep my insulin low, not only because it will slow digestion and prevent an insulin overshoot but also because I'll probably end up eating less glucose overall. And keeping my insulin low is helpful if I'm trying to lose weight, because it will keep my fat cells releasing fat.

Very good.

Gut bacteria II

I'm sorry, but I still don't see what's so special about gut bacteria.

How dare you!

No, I mean, I see why being able to digest fiber is important. But I don't see why it's important that the cells that help me digest fiber happen to be bacteria rather than my own cells. Why does that matter?

It matters because your gut bacteria are born, reproduce and die many times per day, so the makeup of your gut bacteria can change very quickly, much more quickly than the rest of you.

OK, so if I don't eat fiber regularly, my gut bacteria can die out quickly?

Sort of. You'll always have gut bacteria – unless you take antibiotics but we'll get to that later – it's just that, depending on your diet, you'll have more of some kinds of bacteria and less of other kinds. There are bacteria that can take in all of the different things that we eat, so the make-up of your gut bacteria will always reflect the make-up of your diet. If you don't eat fiber, your fiber bacteria will die off and they'll be replaced by other bacteria that take in whatever you do eat. For example, you also have bacteria that help you break down starch. If you eat a lot of starch, you'll have a lot of starch bacteria.

So it's like natural selection in my gut?

That's exactly what it is. In an environment with a lot of fiber, the fiber bacteria will be more likely to survive and reproduce. In an environment with a lot of starch, the starch bacteria will be more likely to survive and reproduce.

OK, so two people with the same diet will have the same gut bacteria?

Not exactly. Like everything else, it's half genetic.[10]

But how can my genes affect which bacteria live in my gut?

Your genes set the general climate of the environment inside your gut and that determines which bacteria will have the best chance of survival. Like the way different trees grow in warm and cold places. Maybe your gut has more acid or less acid than normal or something like that.

But what I eat can still have a big impact, right?

Right. So, actually, that's another good reason to eat fiber. You're better off with a lot of fiber bacteria than, for example, a lot of starch bacteria.

Why?

Because your starch bacteria help you breakdown starch so, if you have more starch bacteria, you'll actually digest more of the starch that you eat.

I'm confused. Don't I always digest all of the starch that I eat?

Oh, no, definitely not. Some of it is just passed out in your feces.

Oh, so my feces isn't just stuff I couldn't digest?

No, no. First of all, half of your feces is bacteria... [11]

Wait, what? Where do they all come from?

I told you, your gut bacteria reproduce very quickly.

Right... OK, so I'm basically like a giant incubator for bacteria?

Pretty much.

OK, go on.

Right, so the other half of your feces includes some food that you could have digested but didn't. After the mush from your stomach enters your intestines, it gets constantly moved along. Whatever you can break down before it gets to the end of your intestines will go into your blood. Whatever makes it to the end of your intestines without getting broken down will be passed out.

I see. So if I have a lot of starch bacteria, they'll help break down the starch I eat so that more of it will get into my blood. If I don't have a lot of starch bacteria, less of the starch that I eat will get broken down and more will get passed out.

Right.

How much does this really matter? I mean, how many calories are we talking about?

A lot. Someone with a lot of starch bacteria and only a few fiber bacteria can easily digest hundreds of calories per day more than someone with a lot of fiber bacteria and only a few starch bacteria, even if they eat exactly the same food.[12]

Why? I mean, I get that the person with a lot of starch bacteria would digest more of the starch. But wouldn't the person with a lot of fiber bacteria digest more of the fiber?

That's right, they would. But you just can't get as many calories out of fiber as you can out of starch, so it doesn't balance out.

OK, so this is yet another obstacle if I'm trying to lose weight. If I gain weight because I am eating a lot of processed foods with no fiber, I'll probably have a lot starch bacteria and I'll actually be getting more calories from my meals than I would otherwise. So I'll need to eat a lot less or exercise a lot more to make up the difference.

Right. But, this time there is a bright side. Remember, the make-up of your gut bacteria can change very quickly, so if you switch from processed foods with no fiber to unprocessed foods with a lot of fiber, your gut bacteria will change to match your new diet[13]: your starch bacteria will die off and your fiber bacteria will survive and reproduce.

Oh, that's good. So then it will be like cutting out hundreds of calories per day, even if I'm eating the exact same food.

Right.

OK, hold on, this sounds too good to be true again. If I start eating a lot of fiber instead of a lot of starch and end up digesting fewer calories because my gut bacteria change, won't my weight regulation systems just find a way to compensate?

Well, again, the answer is maybe. If your weight regulation systems are working properly, then your weight might not change. But if your weight regulation systems aren't working properly, anything

that lowers the number of calories that you take in is going to help, right? But I don't want you to think this is just about fiber versus starch, that's just an example. You have a lot of other gut bacteria that do a lot of important jobs and if you eat unprocessed foods, you can keep them all happy.

What else do my gut bacteria do?

They help breakdown pretty much everything you eat; not just fiber and starch but fat and protein as well. And they make a lot of things that your body needs, like vitamins.

My gut bacteria make vitamins?

Sure. There are even a few vitamins that you can only get from your gut bacteria.[14]

Cool.

And your gut bacteria also do a lot of things that are not related to digestion. Or at least not directly.

Like what?

Well, for starters, it's clear that your gut bacteria have an influence on the signals that your gut sends to your brain.[15] For example, do you remember the hunger hormone ghrelin?

Sure, ghrelin tells my brain how much I've eaten: it's high when my stomach and intestines are empty and it goes down after I eat.

Right. But it turns out that if you eliminate one type of bacteria from your gut, your ghrelin won't go down as much after you eat.[16]

Really?

Yes. And what's interesting is that it happens to be the same type of bacteria that causes ulcers.

I thought ulcers were caused by stress?

No. Stress might play a role but most ulcers are caused by a particular type of bacteria that releases chemicals that damage your stomach or intestinal wall cells. Two guys got the Nobel Prize a few years ago for figuring that out.

Wow. So are ulcers contagious? Can I get these ulcer bacteria from someone else?

Well, most people actually have the ulcer bacteria already. You get your first gut bacteria from your mother when you're born and the rest from the other people that are around you when you're young.

How can bacteria get from one person to another?

Well, it's not really that hard to imagine, is it? When you wipe after going to the bathroom, some of the bacteria that came out in your feces will get on your hand. When you flush the toilet, some of the bacteria will go from your hand to the handle. When the next person flushes…

OK, OK, I get it. So we're all constantly swapping bacteria with each other?

Definitely. But it matters most when we're kids and we're just getting our gut bacteria all set up. Once we're older, the make-up of our gut bacteria usually stays pretty much the same, unless we do something to change it.[17]

Like what?

Well, like we just discussed, the make-up of your gut bacteria will change if you change what you eat. But the really serious changes occur when you take antibiotics.[18]

What happens when I take antibiotics?

Oh, it's like setting off a nuclear bomb in your gut. Most antibiotics kill nearly all bacteria. Usually you take them because you've got dangerous bacteria that you need to get rid of. But they don't just kill the dangerous bacteria, they kill most of your other bacteria as well.

But can't they just make antibiotics that will kill only the dangerous bacteria?

Maybe they will eventually but they haven't yet. Until recently, no one really worried about killing bacteria.

Why not? You said we've known for a long time that we need our gut bacteria to digest fiber.

Right but after you're done with the antibiotics, you'll get new gut bacteria.

How?

From other people, the same way you got them in the first place when you were a kid. They might not be exactly the same ones you had before but they'll probably be similar.[19]

Oh, OK, so the fact that antibiotics kill most of our bacteria isn't really a problem?

Not if you only take antibiotics once in a while. But if you take them all the time, that's a different story. Bacteria have lived in the guts of our animal and human ancestors for millions of years, so we've evolved with them as a part of us.[20] Our bodies expect them to be there and a lot of the things we do depend on interactions with them.

I have to admit, they are pretty cool.

I told you!

OK, so what's next?

Actually, I think we've covered most of the basics now. We've discussed how all of your different metabolic and weight regulation systems work and what can go wrong when they don't work.

Wow. OK, hold on, let me ask you some questions, then.

Sure.

6
Processed foods

Science

OK, first of all, how do you know all this stuff?

I told you, I read all the research studies.

But how do you know that all of this stuff is actually true? I know you're a scientist and I trust that you can understand all of the studies. But aren't the results of studies often wrong or in conflict with each other?

Oh, I see what you're asking. That's a great question. First of all, when it comes to long-term, real-world effects on human health, we can never really know for sure that anything is true.

What do you mean?

The only way to know for sure that something is true is to do a perfect study – a study where there is only one possible explanation for the result – but those studies are impossible to do.

OK, fine. But...

Hold on, I want to make sure that you understand the point that I'm trying to make. If we want to prove something in a lab, we might be able to do a perfect study where we can control all the factors that might influence the result so we can be sure about cause and effect. But we can never do that when we study people in the real world.

OK.

Let's say I wanted to really prove that smoking causes cancer. I'd need to get a large group of young identical twins...

So that you can be sure that genetics don't influence the result?

Right. I'd need to assign one twin from each pair to be the smoker and the other to be the non-smoker for the rest of their lives and ensure that every other thing about their lives was always exactly the same until they died. Then I could compare the number of smokers and non-smokers that got cancer.

OK, I can see how that would be impossible. But why not just bring people into a lab?

Well, we can't really do that for more than a few weeks, right? But, even if we could, there's a trade-off: anytime we do a study in a lab, we can never be sure that the cause and effect would be the same in the real world. For example, I could put some cells into a Petri dish, expose them to the chemicals in cigarettes, and watch them grow tumors. And if the study was perfectly controlled, I could be sure that it was the chemicals that caused the tumors. But I would still have no idea whether the same thing would happen when a person smoked real cigarettes in the real world.

Are you saying you don't believe that smoking causes cancer?

Of course I believe that smoking causes cancer.[1]

Why?

Because there are a lot of studies that are imperfect in different ways that all suggest the same thing. There are many poorly controlled studies of humans that suggest that smokers are more likely to get cancer, there are many well-controlled studies of animals that suggest that cigarette smoke causes cancer and there are many perfectly-controlled studies of cells in a dish that show exactly how the chemicals from cigarettes cause tumors to grow.

But it's impossible to prove.

Right. But just because we can't prove something doesn't mean it isn't true. Like I said, when it comes to human health, it's almost impossible to ever really prove or disprove anything. And you shouldn't necessarily presume that something is false until proven true or vice versa. You should consider all of the evidence and then decide whether or not you believe something, how confident you are in that belief and, most importantly, whether or not it actually matters.

What do you mean?

Well, let's say I did that perfect smoking study with the twins and that the results showed that the smokers are, in fact, more likely to get cancer. And let's say that I had a huge number of twins in the study so I'm absolutely sure that, even if I added more twins, the results wouldn't change – that's called statistical significance. It means that the results are unlikely to be a fluke. Based on those results, I would believe that smoking causes cancer and I'd be extremely confident about that belief.

Right.

But I still haven't told you how much more likely the smokers are to get cancer, so you still don't really know whether you should bother worrying about smoking or not.[2]

Oh, I see. If many more smokers got cancer than non-smokers, then smoking actually matters. But if only a few more smokers got cancer, then smoking doesn't matter.

Exactly. Just because something is statistically significant doesn't mean that it's worth worrying about. If a study is big enough, even a tiny difference between two groups will be statistically significant. But who cares, right? We've got enough to worry about already.

First principles

Right, OK, I'm with you. All of this is fine for something like smoking but what about something that hasn't been studied as much? How do I know what to believe?

Well, in the absence of any studies, you have no choice but to make your best guess based on first principles. If there are a few studies but not many, and they suggest something that goes against first principles, then you have to evaluate how strong the evidence is.

What do you mean by first principles?

I mean simple ideas that can explain a lot.

OK, so what are the first principles that I can use to decide what I should and shouldn't eat?

Why don't you try to tell me?

OK, let's see. One of the main themes so far is the idea that most of our problems are created by the mismatch between the environment that our ancestors evolved in and the environment that we live in today. They evolved in an environment where they had to be active to seek out scarce, unprocessed foods, not an environment where we're constantly surrounded by processed foods or reminders of them.

Right.

If I eat a lot of processed foods, I won't get any fiber, which is a problem for all of the reasons that we just discussed. Processed foods also typically have a lot of added sugar and, therefore, a lot of fructose, which can damage my liver. All that sugar makes processed foods taste too good, so I'm likely to crave them much more than I would crave unprocessed foods. And because processed foods are everywhere, the only way to avoid overeating is to constantly ignore my cravings, which is really hard.

Good.

And I guess the other main theme was inflammation. The mismatch between the environment that our ancestors evolved in and the environment that we live in today might be what causes me to gain weight in the first place but the real problems start once I'm overweight and inflammation has kicked in. It's inflammation, rather than excess body fat itself, that actually causes problems. And it's also inflammation that makes it so hard for me to lose weight once I've gained it.

Right.

If I overeat, my cells won't be able to process all the glucose and fat fast enough, so a lot of waste and half-processed glucose and fat will build up. My immune cells will notice the build-up and start interfering with my insulin, which will prevent more glucose and fat from getting into my cells and give them a chance to clear out the backlog. But if I just keep overeating, I'll be constantly inflamed and my insulin will never work – that's called insulin resistance. My liver will keep making and releasing glucose but my muscles won't use any of it, so I'll end up with high blood glucose and, eventually, diabetes. And my fat cells will keep releasing fat, which my liver will add into the packages that it releases. The extra fat will make the packages smaller after they're depleted and, therefore, more likely to get stuck in my blood vessels. If the depleted liver fat packages start getting stuck faster than my waste packages and immune cells can clear them out, they'll build up into a plaque that'll eventually break off, clog one of my blood vessels and give me a heart attack or a stroke.

Good.

But the real problem is that, even if I want to lose weight, inflammation makes it really difficult because it also interferes with my leptin and causes leptin resistance. Leptin is how my fat cells tell my brain how much fat I have stored. So, normally, if my leptin was high, I would eat less: my leptin would strengthen my gut signals so that I'd feel full after less food, it would interfere with my dopamine to weaken the cravings from my pleasure system and it would strengthen my self-control system so that it could cancel the orders sent by my pleasure system. High leptin would also make me burn more calories: it would make exercise more pleasurable and make me fidget more, and it would let my brain know that it should tell my cells to waste energy by creating heat. But if my brain is inflamed, none of this will happen. In fact, because my leptin isn't working, my brain will actually think that I'm under my natural weight and it will make me eat more and burn fewer calories.

Excellent.

OK, so for first principles, how about "Evolution is good" and "Inflammation is bad."

Ha! Those are pretty good. Let's change "Evolution is good" to "Natural is good." I think it will be more useful that way.

OK.

Actually, hold on, I think "Unprocessed is good" would be even better.

What's the difference?

Well, there are plenty of things that are natural that you don't want to eat a lot of.

Like things that are poisonous?

Oh, sure. But I mean natural things that are added to processed foods.

Oh, like sugar?

Right. There's nothing artificial about sugar. It's not a chemical that's made in a lab, it's just something that is extracted from a plant.

OK. But the amount of sugar in processed foods is artificially high, right?

Right, but I think "Unprocessed is good" covers that. And it also covers all of the other things that are added to processed foods.

Like what?

Oh, there are literally thousands of things that manufacturers are allowed to add to food.[3]

OK, obviously I don't expect you to go through them all. But can you at least give me a few examples?

Additives

Well, some of the most common additives are preservatives.

Right. I know that they make food last longer. But what do they actually do?

They prevent food from changing color or shape or smell, usually by preventing bacteria from growing.

Oh, hold on, swallowing things that prevent bacteria from growing can't be good for my gut bacteria.

Exactly!

Do we know that for sure?

Well, remember, "know" is a strong word. But there is evidence that preservatives are bad for us and, specifically, for our gut bacteria. Should I try to describe a study to you? There was one just recently about the effects of emulsifiers on gut bacteria.[4] Emulsifiers are a very common type of preservative that help keep food smooth and creamy.

OK. But try to keep it simple.

No, don't worry, it's not that complicated. In the first experiment, the researchers split mice into two groups: one group that got normal food and another group that got the same food with added preservatives.

OK. And they controlled all of the other factors so they could be sure that whatever happened was caused by the preservatives, right?

Right.

OK, so what did they find?

They found that the mice that ate the preservatives gained weight and had much higher blood glucose, like people who were on their way to getting diabetes.

Really? Why? Wait, how many preservatives did they give the mice? Was it a lot more than any human would ever eat?

No. But that's a good question. That kind of thing does happen a lot. But in this study they used the same amount of preservatives that we would typically eat in processed foods – adjusted to the smaller size of the mice, of course.

OK, so what happened? Why did the mice that ate the preservatives gain weight?

Well, normally, your intestinal wall cells are covered by a protective layer of mucus. But, when the researchers looked inside the intestines of the mice that ate the preservatives, the mucus layer was gone.

So the preservatives were destroying the mucus?

Not exactly. The researchers did another experiment where they added the preservatives to the food of mice that had no gut bacteria.

How did they get mice without gut bacteria?

They made sure that the mice were born and raised in a sterile lab.

OK, and what happened when the bacteria-free mice ate the preservatives?

Nothing. The preservatives had no effect on the protective mucus layer in the bacteria-free mice.

Really? OK, so I guess the preservatives didn't destroy the mucus directly but they somehow caused gut bacteria to destroy it?

I guess you could say that. There were certainly big differences between the gut bacteria of the mice that ate the preservatives and the mice that didn't.

But can you really be sure that it was the differences in gut bacteria that caused all the problems?

Well, the researchers did another experiment in which they took gut bacteria from the mice that ate the preservatives and put them into the mice that didn't.

That's clever. How did they do that?

Oh, mice will gladly eat each other's feces.

Right. OK, so what happened to the mice that got the new bacteria?

The same thing that happened to the mice that ate the preservatives: they gained weight and their blood glucose went way up.

But those mice never actually ate any of the preservatives, right?

Right. So it really seems like the preservatives changed the gut bacteria, which, in turn, destroyed the protective mucus layer.

Wow, OK. But why would losing the protective mucus layer cause the mice to gain weight and have high blood glucose?

Inflammation!

Of course. It's the leaky gut problem that you were talking about earlier, right? Without the protective mucus layer, things got into their blood that shouldn't have and their immune cells took action. And the chemicals from their immune cells leaked out into other parts of their bodies, interfered with their insulin and so on.

Exactly.

Did the researchers actually measure inflammation? Did they find that there was more inflammation in the mice that ate the preservatives?

Yes. And yes.

OK, that does seem like a pretty good study. But these were mice in a lab and, like you were saying before, we can't be sure that the same thing will happen when real people eat real food in the real world, right?

That's right. And we may never be sure. But, in this case, I don't really care.

Why not?

Because there is no reason to eat preservatives. Why take the risk? If I'm going to eat something that might be bad for me, it should be for a good reason. I know I'm taking a risk when I eat foods with added sugar but sometimes I do it anyway because I like the taste. But that's not true for preservatives. I don't think there is any food that tastes better because it has preservatives. Wouldn't you rather have freshly-baked bread than bread off the grocery store shelf?

Sure, I see what you're saying. But there are a lot of other kinds of additives besides preservatives, right? Some of them must have some potential benefit.

That's right. Artificial sweeteners are a good example. A lot of people drink diet soda to avoid the sugar in regular soda, which makes sense. But it turns out that artificial sweeteners can cause other problems.

Really, like what?

Well, it's not so different from what happens with preservatives: artificial sweeteners can change your gut bacteria, which, in turn, can cause problems with your digestion and metabolism.[5]

Oh, so should I avoid artificial sweeteners?

I think it depends on how much you like them. Personally, I don't like the taste of artificial sweeteners, so I have no reason to eat or drink them. But if I did like their taste, I might use them to help myself eat less actual sugar. If I had trouble resisting my cravings for sweets and I could satisfy them without actually eating any sugar then I might take the risk. But the best thing, of course, would be to avoid food with any added sweeteners – natural or artificial – and eat unprocessed foods that are naturally sweet, like fruit, instead. Fruit has a lot less sugar than processed sweets and it comes along with fiber and other nutrients.

Pesticides

OK, so besides preservatives and artificial sweeteners, are there any other additives that I might want to watch out for?

Like I said, there are all kinds of things that manufacturers are allowed to add to food. When it comes down to it, we don't really know which ones are harmful. I mean, how could we? To get an additive approved, you have to show that when you give large doses of it to animals, nothing obviously terrible happens.[6] Now, that sounds pretty reasonable. But I'm not worried about additives doing something obviously terrible to me, I'm worried about additives making it harder for me to stay lean and healthy. The preservatives and artificial sweeteners that we just discussed were approved because they don't do anything obviously terrible. But it's clear that they're harmful nonetheless – at least to animals.

OK, so your approach is to just avoid additives altogether?

Sure, if I can. What's the downside? OK, it might be more expensive but it doesn't necessarily have to be. And I suppose it can take more time to prepare a meal from unprocessed foods than it does to eat something processed but, well, that's life.

I guess.

Listen, it would be great if healthy eating was as cheap and convenient as unhealthy eating. But it's not. The same way it would be great if I could buy a mansion for the price of a tent or build a mansion in the time it takes to put up a tent. But I can't.

Hey, I'm not trying to argue with you, I'm just trying to figure out what I should eat. I'm OK with the idea that healthy eating might cost a bit more and take a bit more time. But is it really that easy to avoid additives?

Well, you can get a long way by buying unprocessed foods or freshly-prepared foods instead of foods that are processed and packaged to sit on a shelf. If it doesn't have a label with a list of ingredients, it probably doesn't have that many additives.

But even if I buy some raw vegetables, they might have some pesticides or something on them, right?

You're right, that's true. We've talked about things that are added to food when it's processed but there all also plenty of things that are added to food while it's growing. In a sense, pesticides are just like additives: there are a lot of them and we don't really know that much about their long-term effects on humans.

OK...

Wait, actually, that's not quite true. It's obvious that direct exposure to some pesticides is harmful and humans who work with them or near them, such as farm workers, suffer from all kinds of health problems.[7] But is it harmful to eat fruit that still has a small amount of pesticide residue in it? We just don't know. Again, how could we? We can't do a well-controlled study in which we expose humans to chemicals that are known to be harmful – that's not allowed and it's probably unethical. We can't even look for correlations between pesticides and long-term health problems because we really have no accurate way to measure the amount of pesticides that people eat.

OK, so what are we supposed to do?

I'm sorry, I'm not trying to be difficult. I just think it's important to be clear about the fact that there is a lot that we don't know about the things in our food. Maybe there is no reason to worry, maybe all this stuff is fine. Or maybe not. If I wanted to make you think that the pesticides in food are harmful, I could. I could set the whole thing up by telling you how many millions of pounds of pesticides are added to our food each year,[8] and that the pesticides are still there when the food gets to the grocery store.[9] Then I could tug on your heartstrings and tell you that kids are especially vulnerable to pesticides, because their little brains are still developing and their little bodies are too weak to deal with pesticides the way adults can.[10] And then I could top it all off by telling you about a study that found that kids with more pesticides in their urine are more likely to be diagnosed with attention-deficit/hyperactivity disorder (ADHD).[11]

They are?

See! But I'm not going to try to make you think that the pesticides in food are harmful. Nor am I going to try to make you think that the pesticides in food are not harmful. The fact is that there is just very little direct evidence to go on. Without well-controlled studies in which animals are exposed to pesticides in the same way that we would be in the real world, there is really no basis for a strong belief one way or the other.

And studies with humans aren't informative because they are poorly controlled?

Well, there are different kinds of human studies. The best studies are real experiments that try to test whether something has a helpful or harmful effect.

Can you give me an example?

Sure. The studies used for the clinical testing of a new drug are a good example. Those studies usually start by randomly splitting people into two groups: one group that gets the drug being tested and another group that gets only a placebo.

You mean that the second group thinks they are getting the drug but they're really just getting an empty pill or something like that, right?

Right. Assuming the groups are big enough, you can be confident that any difference between the two groups at the end of a study like that was caused by the drug.

But you can never be sure, right? Maybe everyone who got the chemical also decided to take up yoga at the same time.

Sure. But the results of a study like that can still be pretty convincing. On the other hand, studies that just search through existing data to look for correlations are a lot less convincing.

Like the one with the pesticides and the kids with ADHD.

Right. Now, I'm not saying that those kinds of studies are pointless. They can actually be really useful for identifying correlations that can then be studied properly.

What exactly is a correlation?

If two things are correlated, it means that knowing one can help you guess the other. But it doesn't mean that one causes the other. For example, people who live in warmer places are likely to swim more often than people who don't and they're also likely to eat more ice cream. So there's a correlation between how often someone swims and how often they eat ice cream. If you ask me to guess how often someone swims, I'll do better if you first tell me how often they eat ice cream. But you would never think that swimming causes someone to eat ice cream, right?

Got it.

Good. So correlation studies usually aren't very compelling on their own. There was a study a couple of years ago called something like "Does everything we eat cause cancer?"[12] The researchers chose random ingredients from cookbook recipes and then looked for studies involving those ingredients. They found that almost half of the ingredients were correlated with some kind of cancer. Give it a few years and there won't be anything left that we can eat at all!

OK, that's all fine. I can accept that we're really not sure whether pesticides in food are harmful or not and I appreciate that you aren't trying to convince me one way or the other without strong evidence. What I'm more upset about is the idea that pesticides do seem to be harmful to the people who work with them and they might also be harmful to the rest of us, yet there's really no push to cut back on them.

Genetically-modified foods

Well, I think there is a push to cut back on pesticides to some extent. For example, that's one of the motivations for genetically-modified foods.[13]

Oh, right, GM foods. I hear that term a lot but I don't really know what it means.

Well, typically, a genetic modification is the addition of a gene that results in some specific new trait or function.

Yeah, like I said, I don't really know what that means.

Right. OK, well, a gene is a piece of DNA that contains the recipe for a specific chemical. All cells – human, animal, plant, bacteria, etc. – are constantly making chemicals. They do this by following the recipes in their DNA. There are a lot of different factors that determine how much of a particular chemical gets made by a particular cell but, basically, if you add a new recipe into a cell's DNA, it will start making that chemical.

OK, I think I get it. Can you give me an example?

Sure, a good example is GM corn that is pest-resistant. Farmers often have problems with insects eating their corn and, until recently, they would usually try to solve the problem by using pesticides. But now, they can use GM corn to solve the problem.

How?

The GM corn produces its own pesticide.

What? How?

There are bacteria that produce a chemical that is poisonous to insects. Someone took the recipe for that chemical from the DNA of the bacteria and stuck it into the DNA of the corn. Now the corn makes the chemical and, whenever an insect takes a bite of the corn, the insect dies.

Whoa. OK, that's both cool and a little bit crazy. Hold on, how is that any different from using normal pesticides?

Well, I guess in some sense it's not that different. In both cases, we're adding a chemical into our food without really knowing the long-term consequences. But it really does seem like this particular chemical is not harmful to humans at all.[14]

OK, so why all the fuss over GM foods?

Oh, I don't think the fuss is ever really about any specific threat to human health. Some people are just generally opposed to any kind of genetic modification. You know, "Who are we to play God?", "It's a slippery slope," and so on. There are also a lot of specific concerns but they're usually about the effects on the environment.

Like what?

Well, for example, GM corn has been accused of somehow killing bees.[15]

OK...

Well, bees are really important because they help many other plants reproduce – they basically take sperm from one plant and carry it to the eggs of other plants – so killing bees can have knock-on effects on the rest of the environment. But I don't want to get too far off track; let's stick to human health.

Organic foods

OK. Well, anyway, if I want to avoid all of this stuff – additives, pesticides, GM, etc. – I can just eat organic food, right?

Sort of. Organic food is generally free of artificial chemicals but it may still contain natural additives or pesticides.[16] **For example, emulsifiers, the preservatives that we were discussing earlier, are often made from soy and are commonly used in organic foods. And, actually, the bacteria that were used to make the GM corn are often used directly as a pesticide on organic farms. They just spray the bacteria directly on to the plants.**

Um, OK. So is organic food actually any better than non-organic food?

Probably. Even though organic foods might still contain some additives, they typically contain fewer than non-organic foods.

OK. And since there is a lot that we don't know about a lot of additives, we're probably better off eating food that contains fewer of them.

I think so. But this is where a skeptic would say, "But there is no proof that eating organic food is better for you." And they'd be right, there is no proof.[17]

Well, you said that we can never really prove anything when it comes to real-world, long-term effects on human health because we can never do a perfect study. But there might still be strong evidence to support a belief one way or the other.

Oh, right. But, in this case, there is hardly any evidence to consider at all. There just haven't been many studies comparing animals or people who eat organic food and people who don't.

So would you recommend organic food?

I would, yes. But not because I can make a definitive case that organic food is healthier.

So why bother?

Well, in the absence of strong evidence one way or another, what do we do?

We make our best guess based on first principles.

Right. So I tend to eat organic food simply because it tends to be less processed than non-organic food.

7
Interactions between the immune system and gut bacteria

Antibiotics

OK, and what about meat? What does it mean for meat to be organic?

First of all, it means the animals that the meat came from ate only organic food. But it also means that the animals weren't given any growth hormones or antibiotics.

Antibiotics? I can imagine why you would give growth hormones to animals. But why would you give them antibiotics? To keep them from getting sick?

That might be part of it. But it's really for the same reason that you would give them growth hormones: antibiotics make animals bigger.

Really? Like, a lot bigger?

I guess it depends what you mean by a lot but, yeah, something like 10 per cent or 20 per cent.[1]

OK, yeah, that's a lot ... damn.

What?

Well, I thought I was starting to understand everything but this doesn't make any sense to me. Gut bacteria help with digestion so getting rid of them should make it harder to digest food, right? So, if anything, shouldn't animals that take antibiotics be smaller because they are actually digesting fewer calories?

Good! You are getting it! It's true that if you raise animals without any gut bacteria at all, like the bacteria-free mice that we discussed earlier, they end up a lot smaller. That's been demonstrated many times. What I haven't told you is that farm animals are given very low doses of antibiotics – not enough to wipe out all of their gut bacteria but enough so that the animals end up with more of some bacteria and less of others.

I see. So they end up with more of the bacteria that are really helpful for digestion?

That's right.

Do we know that? I mean, are we sure that's why antibiotics make animals bigger? Antibiotics must have all kinds of effects, right?

You're right, there is a bit more to it than just better digestion. There have been a few studies of this recently.[2] Shall I tell you about them?

Please.

OK. First, researchers split mice into two groups at birth: one group that was raised normally and another group that was raised on antibiotics.

Using the same low doses that you would give to farm animals?

Right.

OK, and what happened?

Well, the mice that were on antibiotics gained extra weight, just like the farm animals would.

Right. And were the researchers able to figure out why?

They started by looking at the effects of the antibiotics on gut bacteria. At first glance, the gut bacteria from the two groups of mice weren't all that different.

OK, so the antibiotics weren't wiping out the gut bacteria completely or anything like that?

Right. But when they took a closer look, they did see differences in the relative numbers of certain bacteria.

And were the bacteria from the mice that were on antibiotics better at digestion?

Yes, it seems like they were. When the researchers fed the two groups of mice the same amount of food, they found that the mice that were on antibiotics had fewer calories left in their feces.

OK. And did they do an experiment where they took gut bacteria from mice that were on antibiotics and put them into mice that weren't?

They did.

And?

And the mice that got the new gut bacteria gained extra weight.

Even though they were never on antibiotics themselves?

Right.

OK, so doesn't that settle it?

Not exactly. They also tried giving mice antibiotics for just a short time while they were young. They found that after the mice were taken off the antibiotics, their gut bacteria went back to normal but they still kept gaining extra weight.

Oh. Right, OK, so I guess that means there's more to the story . . . but what?

Well, I mentioned that gut bacteria do a lot of things besides just help with digestion . . .

Right.

One of the other important things that they do – maybe the most important, actually – is control the development of your immune system.[3] So if something happens to your gut bacteria when you're young, your immune system will never work properly, even if your gut bacteria go back to normal when you're older.

Hold on. Are you saying that, in order for my immune system to work properly, I have to have the right gut bacteria?

Yes, that's what I'm saying.

But, why? I mean, doesn't that seem risky? It puts me in such a vulnerable position.

Well, I don't think it was all that risky until recently. There was really no reason that you wouldn't have the right bacteria. It's only nowadays that things have started changing.

If you say so.

OK, you're right that there is some risk in being dependent on bacteria. I'm just saying that the risk is or at least was, relatively small and the benefits are huge.

And what are the benefits exactly?

Evolution

Fast evolution!

Oh, right.

You understand how evolution works, right?

More or less.

Well, it's pretty simple. Whenever we or any other living thing reproduce, our offspring are born with mutations.

You mean our children's DNA is different from ours? Why?

Just because the process of copying DNA isn't perfect. Every time your body makes a copy of your DNA to stick into an egg or a sperm, there are errors – some of the chemical recipes get changed.

OK.

Now, most of the time these errors don't matter at all. But every now and then, one of the mutations will result in a change that is helpful and the offspring that get it will have a better chance of living longer and reproducing more than the rest of the population.

Right.

Good. So then the offspring with the mutation will pass it on to their offspring, who will, in turn, pass it on to their offspring…

Wait, why would the mutation get passed on?

Well, once the mutation happens, it becomes just like any other bit of DNA. There's nothing special about it. It just gets copied and passed on like all the rest.

Oh, OK, sorry – go on.

OK, so the mutation keeps getting passed on and, because it's helpful for survival and reproduction, more and more of the population will end up with the mutation as time goes on.

OK, I'm pretty sure I get it. But can you give me an example?

Sure. The ability to digest milk is a great example. As of 10,000 years ago, no humans could digest milk.[4]

What?

Wait, of course, that's not true – human babies have always been able to digest milk. But adults couldn't.

Why not?

Because milk contains its own kind of sugar called lactose. You need a special enzyme to break it down and, until recently, adults couldn't make it.

What does the enzyme do?

The enzyme breaks lactose into its basic parts, which are glucose, which you already know all about, and galactose, which is found only in milk.

OK. And then the glucose and galactose go from my intestines into my blood just like everything else?

Right.

And what happens to the galactose?

Your liver converts it into glucose.

Is that bad?

No.

OK. But it's bad when my liver converts fructose into glucose or fat, right? How is converting galactose to glucose any different?

Well, it's just a totally different process. Converting fructose into glucose or fat is difficult for your liver cells and produces a lot of waste. Converting galactose into glucose isn't and doesn't.

OK. So what happens if I don't have the enzyme? Is that what it means to be lactose intolerant?

That's right.

So then the lactose just passes right through me?

Nope.

Oh, my gut bacteria digest it, right?

Yup.

And they release gas.

Yup.

Got it. OK, so you're saying that a few thousand years ago, someone was born with a mutation that caused them to keep making the lactose enzyme as an adult.

Right. And remember, at this point, food was still pretty scarce. We'd already begun farming but it wasn't like it is today. So, since milk is a great source of energy and other nutrients, the ability to digest it was a major advantage.

So people with the mutation lived a little longer and reproduced a little more and, as a result, there were more and more of them in every generation.

Exactly. And now, just a few thousand years later, half of us have the mutation.

OK, I get it. So you were saying that the benefit of being dependent on gut bacteria is that this kind of thing can happen much faster?

Right, simply because bacteria reproduce much faster than we do; we might reproduce every 20 years but they reproduce every 20 minutes. And faster reproduction means more chances for mutation. If one of our gut bacteria is born with a mutation that causes it to make a chemical that helps us live longer and reproduce more, it's also going to help the bacteria live longer and reproduce more.

Because we provide them with food and shelter.

Right.

Immune development

OK, so how does it work? I mean, how do my gut bacteria actually control the development of my immune system?

Well, a lot of the details are still being worked out.

OK...

Maybe I should tell you about a few studies.[5]

Yes, please do.

OK, first of all, researchers examined the immune systems of mice with no gut bacteria that were born and raised in a sterile lab.

And these bacteria-free mice are otherwise perfectly normal, right? The only thing that's different about them is that they're born and raised without being exposed to bacteria?

Right. So the bacteria-free mice had an immune system and it kind of worked. But they had the wrong mix of different immune cells.

What do you mean?

There are many different kinds of immune cells that all have different jobs. So if you've got too many of one kind and not enough of another kind, the whole system won't work properly.

I see.

Good. So then the researchers put just one type of bacteria into the guts of the bacteria-free mice right after they were born.

And?

And their immune systems turned out to be relatively normal.

Just from this one type of bacteria?

Right.

OK, hold on. Would this have worked with any bacteria or did they happen to somehow choose the right one?

They chose the right one but for a good reason. We have a lot of this type in our guts and some older studies had already shown that it was somehow communicating with our immune cells.

OK, so somehow the chemical produced by this one type of bacteria made it so that the mice ended up with the right mix of immune cells?

Right. And we can be sure about that because the researchers also did the same experiment with mutant bacteria that couldn't produce the chemical...

You mean they used the same bacteria as before, except that they deleted the recipe for the chemical from the bacteria's DNA?

Right.

And?

And without the chemical, the bacteria had no effect. The mice still had the wrong mix of immune cells.

OK. So did they really need the bacteria at all then? Did they try just giving the chemical to the mice directly?

They did and it worked. The chemical alone was enough to cause the mice to end up with the right mix of immune cells. And the researchers also did a lot of other experiments with the chemical and immune cells in a dish to see exactly how it all worked. But I don't think we need to go into the details.

No, that's fine. OK, so how exactly does this explain what we were talking about before?

I've forgotten what we were talking about before.

You were explaining why low doses of antibiotics make mice keep gaining extra weight, even after they go off the antibiotics and their gut bacteria go back to normal.

Oh, right. Well, the researchers who did those experiments also showed that giving mice low doses of antibiotics had the same kind of effects on the development of their immune system as raising them bacteria-free.

You mean they ended up with the wrong mix of immune cells.

Right. But, actually, there's more to it than that. For your immune system to work properly, it's not enough to just have the right mix of immune cells; those cells also need to learn what they should attack and what they shouldn't.

And gut bacteria are the teachers?

Exactly! In those same experiments we were just talking about, where the researchers found the bacterial chemical that was required for mice to end up with the right mix of immune cells, the researchers also showed that the same chemical was required to prevent the immune cells from attacking harmless bacteria.

But does it really matter whether or not immune cells attack harmless bacteria?

It might. These harmless bacteria might actually have some other important job. And, remember, the chemicals that your immune

cells release when they take action in one part of your body can leak out into other parts of your body and have unintended consequences.

Like interfering with insulin or leptin.

Right. And when your immune system wants to get rid of bacteria in your gut, it can do a lot more than just release a few chemicals.

Like what?

Like give you cramps or diarrhea or make you vomit. Those are all really effective ways to get bacteria out of your gut but they're also pretty miserable. And that's a trade-off you have to make every now and then to protect yourself from something harmful. But if your immune system is constantly trying to get rid of harmless bacteria . . .

Then you spend your life miserable. Does that actually happen to people?

Sure. It's called inflammatory bowel disease (IBD). It affects something like a million people in the US alone.[6]

Yikes. OK. But if it's all down to this one bacterial chemical, can't we just give the chemical to people who need it?

Oh, I didn't really mean to suggest that it's all down to this one chemical, I was just using that as an example. In fact, there are many different bacterial chemicals that are required for your immune system to work properly. For example, do you remember what I said about fiber fat?

I think so. You said that my gut bacteria turn the fiber that I eat into fat and that the cells that make up the walls of my intestines use that fat for energy.

That's right. But fiber fat is important for a lot of other reasons too and one of them is that it helps your immune system work properly.

Really? Yet another reason to eat fiber . . .

Allergies

That's right. It's the same as with the other bacterial chemical that we were just discussing. If you don't get enough fiber fats, you won't end up with the right mix of immune cells.[7] And when you don't have the right mix of immune cells, the cells that you do have will then attack all sorts of things that they shouldn't – not just harmless bacteria but other things as well.

Like what?

Dust, pollen, gluten, nuts…

Hold on, are you saying that the reason that people have all of these allergies nowadays is because they have problems with their gut bacteria?

Well, that is the most likely explanation. But, like most other things related to human health, it's hard to say for sure.

Have there been animal studies showing that disrupting gut bacteria can cause allergies?

Oh, sure. There have been a lot of studies showing that disrupting gut bacteria in mice can cause allergies.[8] If mice are raised bacteria-free or given antibiotics or even just given food without enough fiber, they'll develop allergies that normal mice don't.

But as long as they're given the right gut bacteria or even just the right bacterial chemicals, they'll be fine?

Right. And for a lot of allergies, researchers have even been able to figure out exactly where the interactions between gut bacteria and immune cells are going wrong.

Are you serious? I can't believe I didn't know this.

Oh, it gets even worse. If your immune cells end up really confused, they will even start attacking your other cells. Do you remember the difference between Type 1 diabetes and Type 2 diabetes?

I think so. Type 1 diabetes is the one where you're born with a pancreas that doesn't work and Type 2 diabetes is the one caused by overeating and inflammation.

Sort of. You're not really born with Type 1 diabetes. It does seem that some people are more likely than others to develop Type 1 diabetes because of their genes. But there isn't any one mutation that causes it. Even if one identical twin has it, the other twin probably won't.[9]

Oh. Well, if Type 1 diabetes isn't caused directly by a mutation, then what is it caused by?

Inflammation. If you have Type 1 diabetes, the reason that your pancreas doesn't work is that your immune cells have killed all of your pancreas cells.

Really? Why would they do that? Oh, wait, is it related to gut bacteria?

It does seem like it. Researchers have been able to make mice more or less likely to develop Type 1 diabetes by changing their gut bacteria.[10] Of course, there's no guarantee that the same thing happens in humans. But there is also no reason to think that it doesn't.

Wow. OK, I know that researchers probably can't do experimental studies of the interactions between gut bacteria and immune cells in humans but they can at least do correlation studies, right? Do people with allergies or Type 1 diabetes have different gut bacteria from people who don't?

They do,[11] but the interactions between gut bacteria and immune cells actually go both ways, so it can be hard to know whether gut bacteria are causing problems with immune cells or vice versa.

I'm not sure I understand.

Well, we've talked a lot about how disruptions of your gut bacteria can cause problems with your immune system, right?

Right.

It can also work the other way around. If you have a problem with your immune system, it can cause disruptions in your gut bacteria.

Why?

Because your immune cells are constantly patrolling the walls of your intestines and they have a say over which of your gut bacteria get to stay and which don't.[12]

Oh, so if there is a problem with my immune system, my immune cells might get rid of the wrong bacteria?

Exactly. If your immune cells are having trouble telling apart different bacteria or if they're making and releasing the wrong chemicals, it can cause disruptions in your gut bacteria, which can then, in turn, lead to other problems.[13] So when someone has a problem with their immune system and disrupted gut bacteria, it's hard to know which came first.

OK, this is getting pretty complicated.

Well, that's exactly the point. I really want you to appreciate how complicated the interactions between your gut bacteria and your immune system are and how a small change to either of them can have all kinds of effects.

Leaky gut

OK, well, I think you've definitely made that point. But I still don't see exactly what this has to do with what we were talking about before.

What were we talking about before?

The mice that were given low doses of antibiotics when they were young but then kept gaining extra weight even after their gut bacteria went back to normal.

Oh, right. Well, we know that taking antibiotics will cause a change in your gut bacteria, right?

Right.

And we know a change in your gut bacteria, especially when you're young, can cause problems in your immune system, right?

Right, because your gut bacteria help make sure that you end up with the right mix of immune cells, and they teach those cells what they should and shouldn't attack.

Right. So the reason that the mice raised on antibiotics kept gaining extra weight even after their gut bacteria went back to normal is that their immune systems never went back to normal. The mix of immune cells that you have as an adult, and what they attack and what they don't, is partly determined by the interactions between your gut bacteria and your immune system when you're young. If those interactions go wrong, your immune system might never be normal.

OK, I get that. But how exactly were the problems that these mice had with their immune system causing them to gain extra weight?

Oh, OK, now I understand your question. Right. I guess I haven't explicitly described how problems with your immune system in your gut can cause you to gain weight.

Well, I get that too much inflammation anywhere is generally a bad thing because the chemicals released by immune cells can leak out into other places and interfere with insulin or leptin. But is that all there is to it? Is it just that when I don't have the right gut bacteria and the immune cells in my gut start attacking harmless things, some of the chemicals leak out into the rest of my body and prevent my metabolic and weight regulation systems from working properly?

Sort of. But there's a little more to it than that. It's not just about the immune cells in your gut attacking the wrong things. If you don't have the right gut bacteria and your immune system isn't working properly, your intestinal wall cells will start letting things into your blood that really shouldn't be there. And then, of course, your immune cells will start attacking them.

Oh, right, that's the leaky gut problem you were talking about earlier.

Right. What I said earlier was that you can get a leaky gut if you don't eat enough fiber and your intestinal wall cells don't have enough fiber fats for energy. But that's only part of it. First of all, your intestinal wall cells have a layer of mucus that separates them from your gut bacteria and everything else in your intestines.

Right, you told me about it before when we were talking about preservatives.

Oh, right. So if that mucus layer shrinks or disappears for some reason, it's going to be easier for things to get into your blood.

OK. And when you say "things," what exactly do you mean?

I mean bits of dead bacteria.

Which my immune cells will then attack?

Right.

OK. And if that happens a lot, then the chemicals from my immune cells will leak out into the rest of my body and interfere with my insulin and leptin and so on.

Yeah, that's more or less the idea.

OK, and how do my gut bacteria – I mean, the living ones – fit into all of this?

Your gut bacteria help to make the mucus layer that separates your intestinal wall cells from everything else in your intestines.

Do they make the mucus themselves?

No, you make the mucus. But you won't make it properly if your gut bacteria are not there. Remember the bacteria-free mice that we talked about, the ones raised in a sterile lab?

Sure.

Those mice don't make mucus properly.[14]

I see. So my gut bacteria release a chemical that tells my intestinal wall cells to make the mucus?

That's right.

Why would my gut bacteria want me to make the mucus? Just because it keeps me healthy, which, in turn, keeps them alive and reproducing?

I'm sure that's part of it. But, actually, some of your gut bacteria also eat your mucus and use it for energy.

So these mucus bacteria release a chemical that tells me to make the mucus and then they eat it?

Right, which is great for them and, since having the mucus layer helps keep you healthy, it's also great for you.

OK.

But, again, helping to make the mucus layer is just one example of how your gut bacteria can prevent things from getting into your blood that shouldn't. They also do all kinds of other things, like help make sure that your intestinal wall cells have the right shape and pack themselves together tightly.[15]

OK, I think I get it. If I don't have the right gut bacteria, I'll end up with the wrong mix of immune cells and those cells won't know what they should and shouldn't attack, so they might start attacking harmless things. Also, my mucus layer and my intestinal wall cells won't work properly, so bits of dead bacteria will slip past them into my blood and my immune cells will have to take action.

Right.

And all of this extra inflammation is bad because the chemicals released by my immune cells can leak out into other parts of my body and interfere with my insulin and leptin.

Right.

And when my insulin and leptin aren't working, then my metabolic and weight regulation systems won't work property and I'll have all kinds of problems.

Exactly.

Antibiotics II

OK, so now I think I understand why animals that are raised on antibiotics gain extra weight. But what about people? Are antibiotics making people gain extra weight?

Well, remember, the animals are raised on a constant low dose of antibiotics and, as a result, they always have gut bacteria that are better at digestion and worse at helping their intestines and immune system work properly than their normal gut bacteria would be. But if you take antibiotics, it's going to be a high dose that wipes out most of your bacteria.

Right, but then things will go back to normal when I stop taking the antibiotics, right?

It depends what you mean by "normal." There's no guarantee that you'll end up with exactly the same mix of gut bacteria as you had before but the new mix you end up with won't necessarily be any worse for you.[16] If you take antibiotics once every few years, it's probably no big deal. The problem is that some people take them a lot more frequently than that, especially kids.

Oh, right – and that's especially bad because kids need the right gut bacteria to help their immune system develop properly.

Exactly.

But is there any evidence that people who take a lot of antibiotics actually end up having problems later on?

Oh, sure, there are a lot of correlation studies. For example, one study just came out where researchers compared the medical histories of random people and people who were just diagnosed with diabetes.[17]

Oh, let me guess. They found that the people who became diabetic took a lot more antibiotics before their diagnosis than the random people did during the same time.

That's right.

But that doesn't necessarily mean that the antibiotics caused the diabetes.

No, of course not. But it's consistent with the results of the animal studies that we've been talking about. Now that researchers have recognized the potential problems with antibiotics, they're going

to do a lot more of these correlation studies. We've known for a long time that antibiotics kill bacteria and we understand exactly how they do it. And now we've done all of these well-controlled animal studies that directly link antibiotics to changes in gut bacteria and health problems. If the results of the correlation studies continue to point in the same direction, then the whole chain of evidence will be in place to support a strong belief that heavy use of antibiotics, especially when you're young, may be harmful to your health.

But we can't just stop taking antibiotics, right?

No, we can't. It's a very tricky problem. And, actually, the direct effects of antibiotics on human health that we've been discussing aren't even the main worry. What's really starting to scare people is the rise of antibiotic resistance.[18]

What do you mean?

Bacteria that cannot be killed by antibiotics are becoming much more common.

Why?

Oh, there's nothing complicated about it, it's just evolution. Sometimes bacteria are born with a mutation that makes them resistant to antibiotics. In an environment with a lot of antibiotics, they're obviously going to be a lot more likely to survive and reproduce than normal bacteria. As time goes on, there will be more and more of the resistant bacteria.

OK, that's scary.

It is. But it was always part of the deal. It's the same as any other arms race: we'll keep making better antibiotics and bacteria will keep evolving to be resistant to them. As long as we take the problem seriously, I think we'll be fine. But let's get back to eating.

OK, so what does all of this mean when it comes to eating animals raised on antibiotics? Are the antibiotics still in the meat when it gets to the store?

Yes. But the situation is the same as with pesticides: there really isn't any direct evidence to suggest that eating meat from an animal raised on antibiotics is harmful. It might be, but we just don't know.

So you don't worry about it?

Well, I often eat organic, which, for meat, means that the animals were not raised on antibiotics. But I do it based on first principles rather than because of any specific concerns. And the worries about antibiotic resistance, of course, apply to animals as well. Far more antibiotics are used on animals than are used on people. Do you know how many chickens are killed in the US each day?

Oh, um...no, I have no idea.

23 million![19] Each day! And most of them were raised on antibiotics.

Right. And each of their guts is an environment that encourages the survival of resistant bacteria.

Right. So if you want to eat organic just to avoid contributing to the rise of antibiotic resistance, I think that's reasonable.

OK. But, in general, the message I'm getting is that we really don't know that much about the direct effects of food additives on human health.

Well, we do know that they're very unlikely to immediately kill us.

OK, fine. But, we still don't know that much about their impact on our ability to stay lean and healthy because there simply haven't been that many studies. And even if there have been well-controlled animal studies for some additives, like the preservatives and artificial sweeteners that we discussed, we're still not sure about their impact on humans eating real food in the real world.

That sounds about right. But, again, why not just eat unprocessed foods and avoid additives whenever you can?

Right. It might cost a bit more to buy unprocessed foods but at least I'll be avoiding a lot of potential risks.

Right. Now, of course, not everyone has that option. And if everyone did all of a sudden decide to buy only unprocessed foods without additives, there probably wouldn't be enough food to go around.[20] But those are separate problems.

8
Good and bad fats

Inflammation II

OK. I have to admit, I find it surprising that there have been so few studies of the effects of food on long-term health. Considering how many people have become obese and unhealthy in recent years, shouldn't these studies be a top priority?

Well, we've only been talking about additives. There have been many more studies of food itself. And those studies are, in a sense, much more important: you might be able to avoid additives but you can't avoid food.

Right, I have to eat something.

Right.

OK, so, additives aside, do we know which foods are good for us and which are bad for us?

Well, not exactly. Just because there have been a lot of studies doesn't mean that the results are clear. The perfectly-controlled studies of cells in a dish and the well-controlled animal studies might be clear but often the link to real-world human health is not.

Oh, c'mon. Surely there are some foods that we are pretty sure are good or bad for us, right?

Yes, you're right, there are. Trans fats, for example: everyone agrees that they're bad for us.[1]

Right, you said we would talk about good and bad fats but we never did.

Oh, right, sorry. This is actually a perfect time to do it. It used to be that fats were thought of as good or bad depending on how they affected your "bad cholesterol." Do you remember what "bad cholesterol" is?

It's the depleted liver fat packages right? Because they're the ones that are most likely to get stuck in my blood vessels.

Right. So it used to be that saturated fats, which mostly come from animals, were considered bad because they increased the number of depleted liver fat packages in your blood, and unsaturated fats, which mostly come from fish and plants, were considered good because they didn't.

That sounds reasonable.

Sort of. But, remember, we now know that fat packages are only likely to get stuck in your blood vessels if they end up really small when they're depleted.

Right.

So even if you have a lot of depleted liver fat packages, you're probably fine as long as they don't end up really small.

Right.

Good. So it turns out that, while saturated fats do increase the total number of depleted liver fat packages in your blood, they also make those packages end up *larger* when they're depleted and, therefore, less likely to get stuck in your blood vessels. So in the end, the effects of saturated fats on your liver fat packages might not actually be that bad.[2]

Oh, OK. So there's no such thing as good and bad fats after all?

Hold on, not so fast. Now we know that inflammation is the real problem, so we've started classifying fats as good or bad depending on whether they increase or decrease inflammation.

Can a particular kind of fat really increase or decrease inflammation?

Oh, sure. If you take a dish full of immune cells and drop in different kinds of fats, you will get very different reactions. Some fats will cause immune cells to take action but other fats will calm them down.

Why would immune cells take action against a fat?

Because some fats actually look a lot like bacteria.

What do you mean?

When your immune cells are deciding whether or not to take action against something, they check to see whether it has a chemical pattern they recognize. Some fats have a chemical pattern that looks just like a chemical pattern that is on certain bacteria.

Why? Is that just a coincidence?

Not really. Bacteria are just cells and the walls of all cells are made of fats. So, in order for your immune cells to recognize different bacteria, they need to be able to recognize different fats.

But my blood is full of fats, right?

Right. But when fats are in digested or liver fat packages, your immune cells won't notice them. It's only when fats are in the simple packages released by your fat cells that they might be mistaken for bacteria.

Oh, I see. So that's another reason that insulin resistance is a problem. If my insulin isn't working and my fat cells are constantly releasing fat, there's more of a chance that my immune cells might notice it.

Which will lead to even more inflammation.

Right. OK, so which kinds of fats do immune cells take action against?

Trans fats

Well, like I said, everyone agrees that trans fats are bad for you and one of the reasons is that they cause a lot of inflammation.

And what do trans fats come from, animals or plants?

Neither. We invented them.[3] Trans fats are created by taking unsaturated fats that are normally liquid at room temperature, like vegetable oil, and changing them so that they become solid.

OK, and why would anyone want to do that?

For two reasons. First of all, trans fats are very stable, so if you use them in processed food, the food can be kept on the shelf for ages without any problem. But, more importantly, we actually thought trans fats were healthy, simply because they aren't saturated fats.

But saturated fats aren't even bad, right?

Well, hold on, we're going to come back to saturated fats in a minute. I said that the effects of saturated fats on liver fat packages might not be that bad but there is more to it than that.

Oh, right. Inflammation.

Right. But, anyway, nobody knew any of this 30 or 40 years ago. Back then, everyone thought that saturated fats were bad, so they started replacing them with trans fats.

Can you give me an example?

Sure. I guess one of the most obvious examples was replacing butter with margarine.

Right, OK. But that backfired because trans fats are actually bad for you?

That's right. Trans fats actually do what we used to think saturated fats did.

What do you mean?

We used to think that saturated fats increased our chances of having a heart attack or stroke because of the effect that they had on our depleted liver fat packages. Now we know they don't. But trans fats do.[4]

I see. So eating trans fats will increase the number of small depleted liver fat packages in my blood?

Exactly. And they can also cause inflammation directly. If they're floating around in your blood, your immune cells will notice them and take action.[5]

Got it. So trans fats are bad.

That's right. The whole chain of evidence is in place: the experiments with cells in a dish, the well-controlled animal studies and the human correlation studies all point in the same direction. But trans fats are easy to avoid. If you avoid processed foods, you'll avoid trans fats.

Saturated fats

OK, and I guess you're going to tell me that saturated fats will also get noticed by my immune cells?

That's right.

So saturated fats are bad after all?

Maybe, maybe not. Remember, just because something happens in a dish or in an animal doesn't mean that it will happen in a human eating real food in the real world.

OK, hold on, we need to get into some details here. I eat a lot of meat, so I really need to know whether saturated fats are bad or not.

OK, let me tell you about a few studies.

Yes, please do.

Let's start with what we know from experiments with cells in a dish.[6] Like I said before, if you drop different kinds of fats into a dish full of immune cells, you will get very different reactions. Saturated fats, in particular, evoke a very strong reaction: immune cells attack saturated fats just as if they were harmful bacteria.

OK. And that's because saturated fats have the same chemical pattern as the fats that make up the walls of certain bacteria?

Exactly. And we know this because researchers did the same experiment where they dropped saturated fats into a dish full of immune cells but, instead of using normal immune cells, they used mutant immune cells that had their chemical pattern detectors deactivated.

So when the chemical pattern detectors were deactivated, the immune cells stopped attacking the saturated fats?

Right. But only when one type of detector was deactivated: the detector for the pattern on certain bacteria. When they deactivated the detectors for other patterns, the immune cells still attacked the saturated fats.

OK, so immune cells attack saturated fats because they mistake them for bacteria.

Right. Now, in their next experiment, the researchers added a piece of muscle to the dish.

Why?

To find out whether the inflammation caused by the saturated fats would cause insulin resistance. Do you remember what we said about inflammation interfering with insulin?

Sure, we've been through it a few times now. When my cells are overwhelmed with glucose or fat, a lot of waste and half-processed glucose and fat will build up. My immune cells will notice the build-up and they'll start interfering with my insulin so that my cells have time to clear out the backlog. The chemicals released by my immune cells will interfere with the escort that lets glucose into my cells and prevent my fat cells from storing any more fat.

Right. So in the case of the backlog-driven inflammation, interfering with insulin is the whole point. But the fat-driven inflammation that we've been discussing has nothing do with a build-up of waste or anything like that, it happens because the immune cells mistake fats for bacteria.

I see. So the chemicals released by immune cells when they attack fats may not actually interfere with insulin?

Right, that was something that needed to be tested. So the researchers added a piece of muscle to a dish full of immune cells. Then they added saturated fats and, of course, that caused inflammation. Then they added glucose and insulin to the dish and they found that hardly any of the glucose actually got into the muscle cells.

Could they actually see the chemicals from the immune cells interfering with the insulin?

Yes. I mean, they didn't actually see it with their eyes but they did other tests to be sure about what was going on.

OK. Did they try the same experiment with the mutant immune cells that had their bacterial pattern detector deactivated?

They did. And they found that the glucose got into the muscle cells just fine.

OK. So saturated fats can cause inflammation and that inflammation can cause insulin resistance.

In a dish.

Right; we've still got a long way to go to get to humans eating real food in the real world.

Right. So let's move on to some more realistic experiments in mice.[7] First of all, researchers took mice and injected fat directly into their blood.

Is that really your idea of "more realistic?"

Hey, you asked for details, so I'm taking you through all the different kinds of experiments that have been done.

OK, sorry, go on. So the researchers gave the mice fat injections.

Right; they found that the injections had all the effects on the mice that you'd expect: the mice developed inflammation and insulin resistance and their cells stopped using glucose because the chemicals from their immune cells interfered with their insulin.

But how did the researchers know the inflammation in the mice was caused by their immune cells mistaking fat for bacteria? Couldn't it just be backlog-driven inflammation? If the researchers just kept injecting more and more fat into the mice, their fat cells wouldn't be able to store it all and their immune cells would step in to help them clear out the backlog, right?

Oh, right, sorry. First of all, I should have said that the injection of fat was a one-off and that the researchers only measured the effects in the few hours after the injection. They didn't give the mice weeks of injections to fatten them up or anything like that. But, the real answer to your question is that the researchers also gave fat injections to the mutant mice that had their bacterial pattern detectors deactivated and nothing happened. So the mice didn't develop inflammation and insulin resistance because their fat cells became overwhelmed or because the fat itself was somehow disrupting their metabolic systems. The problem really was that their immune cells were attacking the fat.

But does this really happen when fat enters the blood naturally? If I eat fat, it will enter my blood from my intestines in digested fat packages, so my immune cells won't notice it, right?

That's right. On a meal-by-meal basis, this kind of fat-driven inflammation may not be a problem. But what if you're overweight and the backlog-driven inflammation has kicked in?

Oh, right, then my insulin wouldn't be working and my fat cells would constantly be releasing fat.

Right. And that fat might get noticed by your immune cells.

Which would make them release even more chemicals and make my insulin resistance even worse.

Exactly. And the researchers did an experiment to show that this can actually happen. When they took normal mice and the mutant mice that had their bacterial pattern detectors deactivated and over-fed them for a few months, they found that the normal mice gained much more weight than the mutant mice and also developed more inflammation and insulin resistance.

OK. And both the normal and mutant mice would have had backlog-driven inflammation from overeating but only the normal mice would have had the extra fat-driven inflammation on top of that, right? So any problems that the normal mice had and the mutants didn't had to be caused by the fat-driven inflammation.

That's the idea. Now, before we move on, there's one more study I want to tell you about.[8] We've been talking a lot about body inflammation but it's important to remember that brain inflammation can be just as problematic.

Oh, don't worry, I remember.

Summarize it for me.

If my brain gets inflamed, my leptin won't work properly. As a result, my brain will think that I'm below my natural weight, even if I'm actually above it, so the systems that control how many calories I eat and burn will act to make me gain weight rather than lose it.

Right.

Without leptin to amplify my gut signals, I'll eat more than I should because it will take more food for me to feel full. And without leptin to weaken my pleasure system and strengthen my self-control system, I'll have trouble resisting my cravings.

Good.

I'll also be less active and fidget less. And my brain will tell my cells to save energy when they should be wasting it, so I'll burn fewer calories.

Excellent.

So I guess the same kinds of experiments that have been done to study fat-driven body inflammation have also been done to study fat-driven brain inflammation?

That's right. When researchers took mice and injected saturated fats directly into their brains, they saw the same thing they saw in their bodies: the injections led to inflammation, which caused insulin and leptin resistance.

Because when the chemicals from immune cells interfere with insulin, they also interfere with leptin.

Right.

And the researchers were sure that this was the same kind of fat-driven inflammation? Did they inject fat into the brains of the mutant mice that had their bacterial pattern detectors deactivated?

They did and the injections had no effect on the mutant mice.

OK, OK. I'm willing to believe that saturated fats can cause inflammation. But if fat-driven inflammation really only becomes a problem when my fat cells are constantly releasing fat because I've gained weight and my backlog-driven inflammation is interfering with my insulin, then I can eat saturated fats without any problems as long as I stay lean, right?

Well, not necessarily. It's true that you might not need to worry about the kind of fat-driven inflammation that we've been discussing. But there are other potential problems.

Damn, I knew it sounded too good to be true. OK, keep going.

Leaky gut II

OK, do you remember the leaky gut problem?

I think so. If my intestines aren't working properly, things will get into my blood that really shouldn't be there. I can get a leaky gut if I don't eat enough fiber because my intestinal wall cells won't have enough fiber fats to use for energy. Or, I can also get a leaky gut if the interactions between my gut bacteria and my immune system get disrupted. In that case, the mucus layer that separates my intestinal wall cells from everything else in my intestines might disappear or my intestinal wall cells might not pack themselves tightly enough to keep things from slipping past them.

Good. And do you remember what kinds of things might get into your blood that shouldn't?

Bits of dead bacteria?

That's right. If bits of dead bacteria get into your blood, your immune cells will start attacking them.

Because they can't tell whether the bacteria are alive or dead?

Well, I suppose not. But, dead or alive, you can't really have a lot of bacteria floating around in your blood, right? So, either way, your immune cells need to take action.

Right. And then the chemicals released by my immune cells can leak out into other parts of my body and cause insulin resistance and all of the other problems that come with it.

Exactly. Now, it turns out that bits of dead bacteria can still get into your blood even when your intestines are working properly.

How?

They sneak in as part of digested fat packages.[9]

Ugh. How?

Well, obviously it's not intentional – they're dead, after all. Remember, some bacteria have a chemical pattern that is similar to some of the fats that we eat. So when your intestinal wall cells are making digested fat packages, sometimes they put bits of dead bacteria in by mistake.

And this will happen more often if I eat saturated fats?

That's right.

Because it's saturated fats that have the same chemical pattern as bacteria, so my intestinal wall cells will have trouble telling them apart?

That's the idea.

But how often does this happen? I mean, is this really something I need to worry about?

Should I tell you about some studies?[10]

Yes, please.

OK, so first researchers took normal mice and injected bits of dead bacteria into their blood. As you might expect, they saw that the injections triggered inflammation.

Sure.

Right, not too surprising. So then they kept giving the injections day after day for a few weeks. They found that the mice gained weight and developed insulin resistance and all of the other problems that you would expect.

But that's pretty unrealistic.

It is. But it's also pretty remarkable. The mice were only getting injections of dead bacteria. They weren't getting fat injections or being overfed or anything like that. Yet they still gained weight.

Oh I see. OK, that is remarkable. I guess I'm just getting used to the idea that my weight is going to depend on a lot more than just what I eat. But if you had told me before we started this discussion that bits of dead bacteria in my blood could make me gain weight, I probably would have thought that was crazy.

Me too.

OK, so does this actually happen when bits of dead bacteria get into my blood naturally?

It seems like it. The researchers did another experiment where they just overfed the mice for a few weeks. They found that the overfed mice gained weight, obviously, but they also found that the overfed mice had a lot more dead bacteria in their blood than mice that were fed normally.

Even though the overfed mice weren't actually injected with any dead bacteria?

Right. And they also did another set of experiments with the same mutant mice that we've been talking about.

The mice that had their bacterial pattern detectors deactivated?

Right. Those mice didn't develop any problems after the injections of dead bacteria and they gained a lot less weight when they were overfed.

I see. OK, so the idea is that if I eat a lot of fats, particularly saturated fats, bits of dead bacteria will get put into my digested fat packages. Once those dead bacteria get into my blood, my immune cells will notice them and things will start going downhill from there.

That's right. But there's still a bit more to the story.

Gut bacteria?

Exactly!

I should've known.

It turns out that eating a lot of saturated fat can cause a change in your gut bacteria.

Well, like you said, the make-up of my gut bacteria will always reflect the make-up of my diet.

That's right. But saturated fats, in particular, seem to have a harmful effect. The mix of bacteria that you end up with when you eat a lot of saturated fats can cause you to develop a leaky gut. For example, do you remember the mucus bacteria that I told you about?

I think so. The mucus bacteria release a chemical that tells me to make the mucus layer on my intestines and then they eat some of it, right?

Right. And you won't make the mucus properly unless they tell you to, so having these bacteria in your gut is really important. Without them, you won't have the mucus layer to protect your intestinal wall cells and bits of dead bacteria will be able to get in.

Right. And if I eat a lot of saturated fats, I'll end up with fewer of the mucus bacteria?

That's right. Now, in the last experiment that we discussed, the researchers overfed mice and found that they had a lot more dead bacteria in their blood than mice that were fed normally.

Right. Did the overfed mice also have fewer of the mucus bacteria?

That's right, they did. So the researchers did something very simple: they gave the overfed mice extra mucus bacteria.

And?

And they found giving the overfed mice extra mucus bacteria reduced the amount of dead bacteria in their blood.

OK, well, I'm not surprised that the mucus bacteria helped fix the leaky gut problem – that seems pretty obvious. But how do the researchers know that it was really the saturated fats that were causing the leaky gut problem? Maybe the problem was just that they were overfed in general?

Right. So another group of researchers did a study to show that it really was the saturated fats that were the problem.[11] They split mice into two groups and put them on diets that were the same except for one small difference: one group got saturated fats while the other group got unsaturated fats.

But the total amount of fat was the same for both groups?

That's right.

OK, and what did they find?

The mice that ate the saturated fats gained weight and developed inflammation and insulin resistance but the other mice were fine.

I see. So the problem really was the saturated fats, not just fats in general.

Right. And when the researchers compared the gut bacteria from the two groups of mice, they found a lot of differences. For example, the mice that were eating the saturated fats had a lot fewer of the mucus bacteria.

OK, and did the researchers do the experiment where they put the gut bacteria from one set of mice into the other set of mice?

They did. They took normal mice that were raised on normal food and split them into two groups: one group that got gut bacteria from the mice that were eating the saturated fats and another group that got gut bacteria from the mice that were eating the unsaturated fats. Then the researchers fed both groups of mice saturated fats for a few weeks.

And?

And the mice that got the saturated fat gut bacteria gained more weight and had more inflammation than the mice that got the unsaturated fat gut bacteria.

Even though they ate exactly the same food?

Right.

Summary V

OK, so let me see if I get it.

Go ahead.

When I eat saturated fats, dead bacteria can sneak into my blood along with them in digested fat packages.

Right.

Or the saturated fats can cause a change in my gut bacteria that will leave me with a leaky gut, allowing dead bacteria to get into my blood that way.

Right.

OK. And if dead bacteria start getting into my blood, my immune cells will attack them and release chemicals that can leak out into other parts of my body and start interfering with my insulin.

Right. And once your insulin isn't working...

Then my fat cells will start constantly releasing fat.

Right.

And that can lead to even more inflammation, because my immune cells can mistake some of that fat for bacteria.

Exactly.

OK, I'm confused.

What? No you're not, you just nailed it.

No, I understand the different ways that saturated fats can cause inflammation but I don't see why the mice in these experiments gained weight. I mean, I understand how inflammation can cause me to gain weight in the real world: if inflammation interferes with my insulin and leptin, my brain will think I'm underweight and it will push me to overeat. But these mice couldn't overeat because their eating was controlled, right?

Oh, actually, the mice in these studies could eat as much as they wanted to. But whether they were on the saturated fat diet or the unsaturated fat diet, the total amount that they ate wasn't all that different.

OK, so what happened?

Well, you're right that when your inflammation gets going and your leptin isn't working properly, your brain will make you want to eat more. But that's only half the story, right?

Oh, right. I'll also become less active and burn fewer calories. So is that what happened?

Yup. Actually, in these experiments both groups of mice were similarly active but the mice that were on the saturated fat diet burned a lot fewer calories for the same amount of activity.

And that's because their leptin wasn't working properly, so their brains were telling their cells to save energy when they should have been wasting it, right?

Well, the researchers didn't actually show that. But, yes, I'm sure that was the problem.

Saturated fats II

OK, so what I'm getting from all of this is that I really shouldn't eat saturated fats.

Well, hold on. It's clear that saturated fats can cause inflammation in a lot of different ways, so you probably shouldn't eat a lot of them. And if you're overweight and backlog-driven inflammation has already kicked in, you should really try to avoid them. If I was trying to lose weight, I would try to avoid anything that might increase inflammation.

Right.

So there's no question that saturated fats _can_ cause inflammation. But here's the thing: the diets that the researchers used in these experiments were pretty unrealistic.

What do you mean?

I mean that when the researchers overfed the mice with a lot of fat, they _really_ overfed them with a lot of fat. In some of these experiments, the researchers fed the mice food that was almost 75 per cent fat, which is pretty extreme. Even in these last experiments that we were just discussing, the researchers fed the mice food that was 45 per cent fat, all of which was either saturated or unsaturated.

Those numbers don't really mean much to me.

Well, if you ate only Big Macs ...

Like in _Super Size Me_?

Right, if you ate like the guy in _Super Size Me_, you still wouldn't be eating as much fat as these mice were eating. On the other hand, the researchers have to use such large amounts of fat because they need to be able to see effects within a few weeks or months. It's possible that foods with a lot less saturated fat would have similar effects over the course of several decades.

I see. But there must be studies that have looked at what happens to humans when they eat different fats. I know those studies wouldn't be as well controlled as the animal studies but they still might be able to tell us something, right?

You're right. In fact, there have been quite a few studies but, as we've already discussed, they're often hard to interpret. A human study

can be well-controlled or it can be long but it cannot be both. When it comes to the effects of food on human health, it's really the long-term effects that we're interested in, right? Let's say you kept a group of people in a lab for a month – which would be a very long time for a well-controlled human study – and fed them a lot of saturated fats. And let's say that nothing really happened – no major weight gain or inflammation. What would that tell you?

That eating a lot of saturated fats for one month isn't all that bad for me?

Exactly. But you don't need to decide whether or not to eat saturated fats for one month, you need to decide whether or not to eat them for 1,000 months! Now, if eating something for one month did cause problems, you'd know that you should really avoid it altogether. But the fact that eating something for one month doesn't cause any problems tells you almost nothing.

OK...

So we're left trying to interpret the results of long-term studies, which have other problems. Since long-term studies aren't conducted in a lab, they usually rely on people keeping track of what they eat or, even worse, just trying to remember what they ate when they're asked. Obviously, that isn't going to be very accurate.[12] And there are also all kinds of other factors that can't be controlled. For example, people who eat a lot of saturated fats also seem to smoke more, exercise less and eat less fiber.[13]

But if you have a large enough group of people, can't you factor those other things out somehow?

You can try. But that's a lot easier said than done because it's impossible to know how all of those things interact. Now, having said all of that, we do have one thing going for us.

And what's that?

Trans fats.

Huh?

Well, like I said, it's clear that trans fats are pretty bad for you but, since we only figured that out recently, there were actually several decades during which people were eating a lot of them.

Right. But how does that help?

We can use trans fats as a sort of a model for unhealthy food: they may not be that harmful in the short term but they're likely to cause serious problems in the long term. In fact, even the short-term studies of trans fats almost always found that things were already heading in a bad direction. After a few weeks of eating a lot of trans fats, people would typically have more of the small depleted liver fat packages in their blood – you know, the ones that are likely to get stuck in blood vessels – and they would also have more inflammation. Now, of course, people weren't getting diabetes or having heart attacks after just a few weeks, but the long-term studies of trans fats almost always found strong correlations with serious health problems.

But those studies must have suffered from the same problems as any other studies of human eating, right?

Exactly. But we can use that to our advantage. The trans fats studies tell us what the results of a study *should* look like if something is actually bad for you. When we look at a study of a different kind of fat or any other kind of food, we can try to judge how bad it seems relative to trans fats.

OK, I get it: so we can use trans fats as a kind of benchmark.

Exactly.

OK, so how do saturated fats look relative to trans fats?

Not nearly as bad.[14] Like I said earlier, the effects of saturated fats on all of the different fat packages seems to be neutral. And the associations with inflammation and health problems are there but they're much weaker than for trans fats.

Excellent; so I can eat as much meat as I want!

Well, I wouldn't overdo it. While parts of the animal studies that we discussed might be a bit unrealistic, I think there is still enough evidence to suggest that when it comes to saturated fats you should proceed with caution. Plus, there is more to meat than just saturated fat.

Oh, no, please don't. Actually, you know what, I've gotta go. I just remembered that I have an appointment.

Oh, c'mon, don't worry. I'm not going to tell you that you should stop eating meat altogether. But there are a few other things to consider.

Fine, go on.

Science II

It turns out that meats, especially red meats, have certain chemicals in them that can be problematic.

Do you mean added chemicals or chemicals that are in the meat naturally?

Oh, I mean chemicals that are in the meat naturally. But, of course, there are added chemicals that are problematic as well. For example, there are preservatives called nitrates that are used in a lot of processed meats, like cold cuts or sausages. I was actually reading about them the other day. They haven't really been studied that much but there's a fair amount of evidence suggesting that they're harmful. Personally, from a decision-making standpoint, I don't care: I avoid processed foods, so I don't need to worry about nitrates. But I still found it interesting to read about them. I came across one study[15] that started with a summary paragraph saying something like "Nitrates are totally fine, nothing to worry about." I thought that was strange, so I skipped to the end of the study where the conflicts of interest are mentioned and it said something like "The researchers who did this study own a company that sells nitrates" and "This study was funded by the American Meat Association." What a joke! I mean, how am I supposed to believe anything those researchers say?

I see the problem. But you're a scientist. You can read the study and decide for yourself whether to believe it or not, right?

Oh. Right. I can see why you would think that, but that's not really how it works. Hmm... I think it's time for me to come clean about something.

What?

Well, you see, the thing is that science is *very* complicated. So complicated, in fact, that it's often hard for scientists to identify the problems with studies in their own field, let alone in a different field.

What do you mean?

Let me give you an example. I told you that when researchers put saturated fats into a dish full of immune cells, the immune cells attacked the fats.

Right.

Well, that is, in fact, true. But, a few years after that first experiment, other researchers started asking questions about whether it was really the fats themselves that the immune cells were attacking.[16] It turns out that when the researchers made the saturated fat mixture, they also used another chemical that could cause inflammation. In the end, they did more experiments without the other chemical to prove that their original conclusion was correct.[17] But, unless you're someone who has experience making fat mixtures, you'd never even know to ask about the other chemicals that were used. The problem is that every experiment involves dozens of little details like that and only people who have done similar experiments themselves would know to ask about them.

OK. You're a neuroscientist, so you study the brain. Are you saying that you don't really have the knowledge or experience to judge the quality of a study about immune cells or gut bacteria?

Yes, that's what I'm saying. I mean, I know *bad* science when I see it. Logical flaws, too few data points, bad statistics – you don't need to be an expert in a field to notice things like that. But am I qualified to evaluate every detail of an experiment outside of my field? No, I'm not. And do those details matter? Yes, they do.

OK, so, not to be rude or anything, but why am I listening to you, then?

That's a fair question. But think about all of the things that we've talked about: metabolism, digestion, hormones, inflammation, brain function, stress, gut bacteria, food, exercise and so on – *nobody* is an expert on all of those things or even most of those things. But if you really want to understand how eating affects your health, you have to consider all of those things and understand how they all fit together.

OK, I see the problem. But then how can I trust you or anyone else to be giving me the right information? Maybe there are problems with some of the studies we've been discussing that you haven't noticed?

That's entirely possible and you certainly shouldn't trust any one person to be your only source of information on any topic as wide ranging as this one. It would be great if a group of experts that could cover all of the relevant topics got together and wrote a book that non-scientists could understand, but that hasn't happened. There are some very good books by experts on specific topics and some of them are actually pretty readable. But, unless you can already see the big picture, it's difficult to see how all of the information in those different books fits together. Now, my hope is that when we're done here, you'll not only see the big picture but you'll also feel like you have a good understanding of the important details. Even if you're not fully convinced by what I've told you and you decide you want more details, you should know enough to go off and read some of the other books or even the original research studies.

But would there really be any point in that? I mean, how am I supposed to judge the quality of studies if you can't?

That's a good question. First of all, if the researchers who did a study had a direct financial conflict of interest – like the nitrate salesmen I mentioned earlier – you should just ignore it entirely. Experts in the field might be able to judge how serious the conflict is and whether they should believe the results of the study or not. But you'll never be able to judge that yourself. If the results of a study are correct and important, they'll be replicated in other studies that don't have any conflicts, so you'll find out about them eventually.

OK, that sounds simple enough.

Now, I don't mean to suggest that financial conflicts of interest are the only kind. Even "pure" academic researchers have their problems: maybe they have a pet theory that they really want to prove or they've spent decades arguing in support of something and it's too late for them to backtrack now. There isn't much you can do about that kind of stuff. But, on the other hand, it's not something that I really worry about.

Why not?

Well, while you may want to be careful not to put too much trust in any one scientist, I think you can safely put a lot of trust in science itself. If a field is large enough – and many of those that we've been discussing involve thousands of researchers – no one group of researchers is going to be able to control it. Given enough time, scientists will always converge on a solid, evidence-based consensus on any important topic.

So says the scientist.

Oh, c'mon.

No, I'm happy to believe that science does generally come up with the right answers in the end, but how do I know what to think about any one study? Let's a say a new study comes out and it says something controversial, how do I know if I should believe it?

Well, the best thing to do would be to ask an expert in the field.

Oh, yeah, sure, hold on, let me get my Rolodex out.

OK, well, I think the best thing to do is just wait a few years for scientists to reach a consensus. Scientists are constantly publishing reviews that summarize the consensus in a field. If you're not an expert, you're better off ignoring individual studies and just focusing on those reviews.

But that means I'm always going to be a few years behind, right?

Does that really matter? Let's assume that your diet is already a reasonable mix of mostly unprocessed foods. What kind of study could come out that would cause you to make an immediate and substantial change to what you eat? There's never going to be a study that says "Actually, you know what, we just figured out that eating garlic will kill you." What you want to keep track of is, for example, how the consensus regarding saturated fats changes over time. Maybe over the next 10 years, scientists will be able to say "Yes, we are now pretty sure that eating a lot of saturated fats causes inflammation even in lean people." Then you'll know that you should really try to avoid them – or maybe they'll say the opposite. Then you'll know that you can eat them without worrying. In the meantime, just make sure to eat a lot of different unprocessed foods to hedge your bets and you'll probably be fine.

Red meat

But not too much red meat?

Well, there do seem to be chemicals in red meat that have the potential to cause problems.

What kind of problems?

Oh, a lot of different kinds. There have been a few recent animal studies[18] showing how chemicals from red meat can cause inflammation or lead to a leaky gut the same way that saturated fats can. But, even though these studies were well controlled and clearly demonstrate that chemicals from red meat *can* be harmful, they were also pretty

unrealistic. So it's impossible to say at the moment whether or not you would have problems if you ate a lot of red meat.

OK, so do I really need to worry?

Well, there's another way that red meat can cause problems. There are chemicals in red meat that can be harmful because of a particular effect they have on your immune cells. They make your immune cells more likely to take action against depleted liver fat packages that are stuck in your blood vessels but less likely to actually break them up. So the plaques in your blood vessels grow faster and end up bigger than they would otherwise, which makes it more likely that one of them will break off and cause a heart attack or a stroke[19].

Yikes. And how much red meat do I need to eat for this to happen?

Exactly 6.25 ounces per week.

What? Oh, c'mon, I wasn't suggesting there is some magic number, I just want to know how much I should worry. Like I said, I really like meat.

I know, I was just kidding. As with everything else, it's very hard to say how much is too much when it comes to humans eating real food in the real world. But I can tell you about a few studies[20] that might help you understand the problem a bit better.

Yes, please do.

OK, the first thing you need to know is that your gut bacteria play a critical role in digesting red meat.

Of course they do.

Researchers fed red meat chemicals to normal mice...

Wait, they just fed them the chemicals, not the meat itself?

That's right, but don't worry, we'll get to more realistic studies in a minute. So when they fed red meat chemicals to normal mice, they found that the mice ended up with a lot of the harmful chemicals in their blood. But when they fed the same red meat chemicals to bacteria-free mice, the bacteria-free mice didn't end up with any of the harmful chemicals in their blood.

Oh, so the mice couldn't digest the harmful red meat chemicals without gut bacteria?

Sort of. It's really that certain gut bacteria change the chemicals to make them harmful. If the chemicals just stayed the way they were in the meat, they actually wouldn't be harmful: they only become harmful after gut bacteria get hold of them and change them.

OK, so what's the upside here? I mean, why would evolution leave me with gut bacteria that change harmless chemicals into harmful ones?

Well, you actually need some of these red meat chemicals to survive. It's only in large quantities that they become harmful.

So how do vegetarians survive?

Oh, the chemicals aren't only found in red meat. Red meat just has more of them than other foods.[21] And, of course, we are eating way more red meat now than our ancestors would have, so it's only recently that we would have any reason to worry.

OK, so mice without gut bacteria don't end up with harmful red meat chemicals in their blood.

That's right. And the same is true of humans. The same researchers fed red meat to humans that were on antibiotics and they didn't end up with any of the harmful chemicals in their blood either.

Oh, I see. And are we sure that having more of these chemicals in your blood is actually harmful?

Yeah, we're pretty sure. The researchers did another experiment with mutant mice that had a mutation in their liver that prevented them from recycling their depleted fat packages.

So the depleted fat packages just kept floating around in their blood?

Right, so these mutant mice end up with a lot of plaques in their blood vessels even when they just eat normal food. But when the researchers fed the red meat chemicals to these mice, they ended up with twice as many plaques as they normally do.

And did they give antibiotics to these mutant mice?

They did. And they found that giving them antibiotics reduced the number of plaques in their blood vessels. After the antibiotics, the mutant mice that were eating the red meat chemicals had the same number of plaques as the mutant mice that were eating normal food.

OK, listen, I'll admit that these are interesting experiments, but you're going to have to do better than red meat chemicals and mutant mice if you expect me to cut back on steak.

OK, hold on, there are few more experiments I want to tell you about. First of all, researchers took blood samples from two groups of humans – vegetarians and meat eaters – and they found that the meat eaters had a lot of the harmful red meat chemicals floating around in their blood but the vegetarians didn't.

I guess that's not too surprising.

No. But then the researchers fed the two groups of people the same amount of red meat chemicals. They found that the meat eaters ended up with the harmful chemicals in their blood, which, again, is not too surprising. But they also found that the vegetarians didn't, which is surprising.

You mean that, even though the vegetarians ate the red meat chemicals, they didn't end up with any of the harmful chemicals in their blood?

Right.

Were they on antibiotics or something?

Nope.

OK, so what happened?

Well, it's just another example of how your gut bacteria will adapt to your diet. If you stop eating meat, then bacteria that digest meat won't be able to survive in your gut, right? Instead, they'll be replaced by other bacteria that digest fiber or whatever it is that you do eat.[22] Once that happens, even if you do start eating meat again, you won't have any of the bacteria that change the red meat chemicals into their harmful form.

Oh, right, I see. But that wouldn't last, right? If I went back to eating meat, wouldn't the meat bacteria eventually come back?

That's right, they would, because you're constantly exposed to bacteria from other people. If some meat bacteria from other people happen to get into your gut, and you've started eating meat again, those bacteria will be able to survive and reproduce.

Got it.

Good, because I think this is a really key point. Your gut bacteria are always going to amplify the effects of the food that you eat.[23] If you eat a lot of meat, you'll end up with a lot of meat bacteria and, therefore, a lot of harmful chemicals in your blood every time you eat meat. So if you eat a lot of meat and I don't, then you're going to get more harmful chemicals from the same piece of steak than I will, right?

Right, I'm with you. But if it's so important to have the right mix of gut bacteria, why don't doctors do gut bacteria transfers between people? You know, like researchers do with mice?

Now you're talking. I'm sure that will become common practice in the future. But it isn't yet.[24]

Why not?

Because there's still a lot that we don't know. We still don't know what the best mix of gut bacteria is in general, let alone for individual people with specific problems. And we still don't really know how to actually make a transfer work.

What do you mean?

Well, it's easy enough to get bacteria into your gut one way or another. But there is no guarantee that they will survive. That's going to depend a lot on the environment inside your gut. So it's not just about giving you the right bacteria, it's also about changing the environment inside your gut so that they can survive.[25]

I see.

And, of course, there's no point in giving you the right bacteria if you're not going to feed them properly. You could get a transfer to replace meat bacteria with fiber bacteria,[26] but if you're just going to keep eating a lot of meat and very little fiber, then you're just going to end up back where you started anyway.

Right.

So all you can really do at the moment is try to eat a mix of different unprocessed foods: at least that will prevent your gut bacteria from getting too specialized one way or the other. Maybe there is a particular set of gut bacteria that is best for you but there is no way of knowing that at the moment, so you should probably just hedge your bets and play it safe. There have been a number of studies showing that healthy people have a much larger mix of different types of gut bacteria than unhealthy people.[27] Now, that could be for any number of reasons but it does reinforce the idea that it's good to have a mix of different gut bacteria and, therefore, to eat a mix of different foods.

Sure, that makes sense. But a mix of different foods could include red meat several times per week or it could include red meat several times per month. I'd prefer to eat it several times per week but, from what you've told me, I still don't know whether or not that is a bad idea. It's great that researchers have figured out how gut bacteria can change red meat chemicals in a way that can lead to more plaques but, well...

Just because we know a lot about something doesn't mean that it's important?

Exactly.

You're right, and I can see how you might find all of this a bit unsatisfying. But there is a fundamental problem that we simply cannot overcome: we want to know the long-term effects of different foods on human health, but we cannot do controlled studies to test them. So when it comes to deciding exactly which mix of foods to eat, we're left with no choice but to guess. I'd love to be able to tell you exactly how much red meat you should eat per week but I just can't. Here's what I can tell you: there's a well-understood way in which the chemicals in red meat can cause problems in animals and there's a strong correlation between how much of these red meat chemicals humans have in their blood and how likely they are to have a heart attack or a stroke.[28]

Oh, you didn't tell me that last part before. Is the correlation in humans stronger than it is for trans fats?

Oh, much stronger.

Oh, so doesn't that mean that I should really try to avoid red meat, then?

Not necessarily. It's not fair to compare the risk associated with having something in your blood to the risk associated with eating something, because not all of what you eat will actually get into your blood. It seems pretty clear that having a lot of these red meat chemicals in your blood is bad for you but it's not clear how much the amount of these chemicals in your blood actually depends on what you eat.

Oh, right – like cholesterol.

Right: if you eat a lot of cholesterol, your body will make less. If you only eat a little cholesterol, your body will make more. Now, these red meat chemicals are different from cholesterol because we can't make them ourselves. But maybe some people are better at digesting the chemicals than other people or worse at clearing the chemicals out of their blood and into their urine. Those people might have a lot of the chemicals in their blood even if they don't eat a lot of meat. The problem is that when you look directly at the correlation between how much red meat people eat and how likely they are to have a heart attack or a stroke, it's much, much weaker.[29]

How weak?

Well, the studies usually conclude by saying something like "If an average person ate an extra serving of red meat per day, their chance of having a heart attack or a stroke would increase by 10 per cent."

Oh, only a 10 per cent increase for an extra serving of meat every day? That doesn't sound that bad after all.

No, it doesn't. But, remember, these correlation studies are based on information that can be very inaccurate. And the risk associated with that inaccuracy runs both ways: not only can it make it seem like there's a correlation between two things when there really isn't, it can also mask a correlation that is, in fact, really strong.

Right.

So here's what I'm willing to say: eating red meat several times per month is probably fine but eating it several times per week might not be. That's as far as you'll get me to go. Personally, given all of the evidence, I'd keep it to a few times per month.

OK, fine. But what should I eat then? You've told me about a lot of things that I shouldn't eat. I'm not sure what's left.

Oh, stop it. What have I really told you not to eat? I've said that you should avoid processed foods. Beyond that, I've suggested that maybe you should go easy on saturated fats, especially red meat. If you think that leaves you with nothing left to eat, you've really got the wrong idea about food.

OK, then tell me something I can eat a lot of.

Vegetables.

Right. Vegetables are great and all, but I can tell you right now that I would get bored of them pretty quickly.

Well, I'm not saying you should eat only vegetables, but if you want to be healthy, vegetables need to be a big part of your diet. You're going to have to come to terms with that sooner or later. But what about fish?

Fish fats

I like fish.

Good, because there is a specific type of unsaturated fat in fish that actually seems to be good for you.[30]

Why would fish fats be good for me?

Well, do you remember what we said about saturated fats?

Sure. The problem with saturated fats is that they can cause inflammation.

How?

There are a few different ways. Saturated fats look a lot like a certain kind of bacteria, so my immune cells might take action against them directly.

Right.

Or they can cause inflammation indirectly by making it so that dead bacteria get into my blood.

How?

When my intestinal wall cells are making digested fat packages with saturated fats, they might put in some dead bacteria by mistake.

Or?

Or saturated fats can change my gut bacteria in a way that leaves me with a leaky gut, so dead bacteria can get into my blood that way.

Right. Now, the exact opposite of what you just said about saturated fats seems to be true about fish fats.

Do you mean that fish fats actually decrease inflammation?

That's right.

How?

Normally, when something is in your blood that shouldn't be there, your immune cells will recognize it with one of their pattern detectors and release chemicals to deal with it. Fish fats stop those chemicals from being released.[31]

How?

Your immune cells also have a pattern detector that can recognize fish fats. When that detector is activated, it prevents the immune cells from releasing chemicals.

Why?

Well, when GPR120 couples with β-arrestin-2 and is internalized, it prevents the association of TAB1 with TAK1, which in turn prevents downstream signaling to IKKβ/NFkB and JNK1/AP1.[32]

What? OK, first of all, I want you to promise to never say anything like that again. Second of all, you misunderstood my question. Why would fish fat prevent immune cells from releasing chemicals? I mean, what's the point? Surely this isn't some elaborate scheme that evolution concocted in anticipation of a day when we would need to decrease our inflammation by eating a lot of fish...

Oh. That's a good question. Just like with saturated fats, it seems to be a case of mistaken identity. Fish fats actually look a lot like another chemical that your body uses to decrease inflammation.[33] The same way saturated fats can increase inflammation because immune cells mistake them for bacteria, fish fats can decrease inflammation because immune cells mistake them for this other chemical.

I see. OK, so does this really work? I mean, should I be eating a lot of fish for this reason?

Maybe.

Arrgh!

Let me tell you about a few studies.[34]

OK, go ahead.

OK, first of all, do you remember the experiments I told you about where the researchers dropped saturated fats into a dish full of immune cells?

I think so. The immune cells attack the saturated fats, right?

Right. But when they dropped fish fats into the dish at the same time, it stopped the immune cells from attacking the saturated fats.

I see.

And they did the same experiment with mutant immune cells that had their fish fat pattern detectors deactivated.

Let me guess: because the mutant immune cells couldn't detect the fish fats, they kept attacking the saturated fats even when the researchers dropped fish fats into the dish at the same time?

Right. So then the researchers did another set of experiments. First, they overfed normal mice with a lot of fat – not fish fats but a mix of other fats – and the mice gained weight and developed inflammation and insulin resistance.

Sure.

Then the researchers split the mice into two groups: one group that they kept overfeeding as before and another group that got fish fats instead of some of the other fats.

And?

And the group that got the fish fats stopped gaining weight and their inflammation and insulin resistance decreased.

Right. And then they did the same experiment with the mutant mice that had their fish fat pattern detectors deactivated, right?

Right. And?

And the effect of the fish fats went away. It didn't matter whether or not the mutant mice got the fish fats because their immune cells couldn't detect them, so they had similar weight gain, inflammation and insulin resistance either way.

Very good. Then what?

Well, maybe they checked whether fish fats decreased brain inflammation as well?

That's right, they did. They found that brain immune cells have the same fish fat pattern detector as body immune cells and when they injected fish fats into the brains of the normal mice that they were overfeeding, the mice started eating less and losing weight.

And that's because the fish fats decreased the inflammation and leptin resistance in their brains.

Exactly.

OK, then they must have also done some experiments to see if gut bacteria were involved, right?

That's right. I'll spare you the details but you can imagine what the results were, right?

I assume that fish fats had the opposite effect of saturated fats.

Meaning?

Meaning that fish fats had a positive effect on gut bacteria and helped prevent a leaky gut.

That's right. For example, when they fed mice a lot of fish fats, the mice ended up with more of the mucus bacteria that tell intestinal wall cells to make the protective mucus layer.

Right. OK, so, again, we have a good understanding of how fish fats *can* decrease inflammation in a dish and in animals. But what about in humans eating real food in the real world?

Well, there is evidence that people who eat a lot of fish fats are less likely to have a heart attack or a stroke, but it's pretty weak.[35]

But the effects in the animal studies were really strong, right? So what's the problem? Is it that the human studies were poorly controlled or that the animal studies used unrealistic amounts of fish fat?

A bit of both. And you have to remember that humans are not animals. It's entirely possible that something could have a strong effect in an animal but not in a human.[36]

Why?

Well, there are differences between animal immune cells and human immune cells. The differences appear to be pretty minor but they could still be important. For example, mouse immune cells are better at detecting fish fats than human immune cells are.[37]

Oh, so does that explain why the mouse studies found strong effects and the human studies didn't'?

That might be part of it, but it's very hard to know.

OK. Listen, I'm pretty sure I've followed most of what you've said, but these experiments are all starting to sound the same to me. It seems like if I want to know whether a particular food is healthy or unhealthy, what I really need to know is how that food affects my immune system and my gut bacteria.

That's exactly right. But I would add one more thing: if you want to know whether a particular food is healthy or unhealthy, you also need to know how eating that food will affect your eating in the future.

What do you mean?

Well, we've just spent a lot time discussing how inflammation can be caused by specific foods, but you shouldn't forget about backlog-driven inflammation. The worst kind of food is too much food. The surest way to get your inflammation going is to overeat.

So you're saying that if I want to know whether a particular food is healthy or unhealthy, I need to know how it affects my immune system and my gut bacteria but also how much it encourages overeating?

Exactly.

9
Sugar and drinks

Fructose II

And that brings us back to the one thing that you should worry about more than any other: sugar. Sugar ticks all of the unhealthy boxes: it causes inflammation, it disrupts your gut bacteria and it promotes overeating.[1]

OK. Do you want to tell me about some experiments?

I could, but I'm not sure it would be that helpful. It's all the same stuff you've heard before: mutant mice, leaky guts, pattern detectors, antibiotics, gut bacteria swaps.[2] The bottom line is that the fructose in sugar can disrupt your gut bacteria and cause inflammation.

OK, yeah, I suppose there's no point in going through the experiments if they're just the same as all of the others.

Good. But what makes fructose even worse than all of the other things that disrupt gut bacteria and cause inflammation is the additional effects it can have on your liver.

Right. Because my other cells can't really use fructose for energy, so it all has to get processed in my liver.

Right. And the parts of your liver that process fructose simply aren't designed for heavy use. A small amount of fructose is fine. But the huge amounts that are in processed foods with added sugar are dangerous.

But fruits also have fructose, right?

Yes, but not enough to worry about. What's your favorite fruit?

Um, probably raspberries.

OK. A large coke from McDonald's has 50 grams of fructose.[3] Do you know how many raspberries you have to eat to get 50 grams of fructose?

I'm sorry, I don't know. I have no intuition for things like that.

1,000!

What?

You heard me. You have to eat 1,000 raspberries to the get the same amount of fructose that you get from a large coke.[4]

Oh.

Right. Now, the problem is that when you eat processed foods that have a lot of sugar and your liver has to process it all, a huge amount of waste is created. And that gets the attention of your immune cells.

So what you're saying is that fructose causes backlog-driven inflammation much more easily than glucose or fat would, right?

Right. And your liver is a particularly bad place to have inflammation and insulin resistance. Do you remember what insulin does in your liver?

It tells my liver to stop making and releasing glucose, right?

Right. When you're between meals and your blood glucose and insulin are low, your liver will make and release glucose to keep your brain going. But if you've just eaten a lot of glucose, your insulin will go up and your liver will know that it can stop making and releasing glucose for a while.

Right. But if I have inflammation in my liver and my insulin isn't working, it'll just keep making and releasing glucose all the time – glucose I don't actually need.

Right, which means that your blood glucose will always be high. And if you also have inflammation and insulin resistance in the rest of your body, then none of that glucose will be able to get into your cells. It will just keep floating around in your blood.

And that's diabetes, right?

Right.

OK, got it.

Good. And do you remember what your liver actually does with fructose?

It converts it to either glucose or fat, right?

Right. And it usually chooses fat. Now, that isn't necessarily a problem, but it can become one. Having a lot of fat in your liver is not a good thing.

Right, because my liver will put the fat into the packages it releases into my blood. And if those packages start off with a lot of fat in them, they'll end up smaller when they're depleted. And small depleted liver fat packages are the ones that are likely to get stuck in my blood vessels, cause a plaque to build up and give me a heart attack or a stroke.

Exactly. And if you're eating so much fructose that your liver can't package all of the fat quickly enough, the fat will build up in your liver and prevent it from functioning properly. That's fatty liver disease.

Right. OK, so if there's one thing I should really try to cut down on, it's sugar.

Right. But, of course, that's a lot easier said than done.

Because sugar tastes so good.

That's definitely a big part of it, but there's more to it as well. Do you remember all of the signals that your brain monitors in order to decide when to make you feel full?

Oh, I don't know: let's see. The hunger cells in my hypothalamus monitor my gut signals, like the hunger hormone ghrelin, to know how much food is in my stomach and intestines and what's coming into my blood.

Right.

And it also monitors how much insulin, glucose and fat are in my blood.

Right.

And, of course, it monitors my leptin to know how much fat I have stored.

Good. Another one of the many problems with fructose is that it has no effect on any of those signals, at least not right away: it doesn't

decrease ghrelin, it doesn't increase the amount of insulin, glucose or fat in your blood and it doesn't increase leptin.[5]

Hold on, hold on. Let's take those one at a time. Why doesn't fructose increase ghrelin?

Because the cells in your gut that release ghrelin don't notice fructose. They don't have a detector for it. I mean, why would they? Until recently, fructose didn't matter.

What do you mean?

Until recently, our ancestors ate only unprocessed foods, right?

Right.

Well, that means that they weren't getting many calories from fructose, so they never developed a way to count them. Even if one of our ancestors had been born with a mutation that allowed them to count the calories in fructose, the mutation wouldn't have become common because it wouldn't have been that helpful.

Oh, right. OK.

And fructose doesn't increase the amount of insulin, glucose or fat in your blood because, well, it's not glucose or fat. It will get converted to glucose or fat eventually but not in time to make you feel full from your current meal.

OK. But I don't understand why you would say that fructose doesn't increase leptin. I mean, if fructose gets converted to fat and that fat gets stored in my fat cells, then my leptin will go up, right?

Oh, right. It's true that whether your leptin is high or low depends mostly on how much fat you have stored, but it also fluctuates throughout the day as you eat.[6] Eating glucose, for example, will increase your leptin temporarily. But eating fructose will not.

Oh, I see. OK, I think I get it. When I eat glucose and fat, my ghrelin goes down, the amount of insulin, glucose and fat in my blood goes up and my leptin goes up, at least a bit. And when my brain notices all of these signals, it makes me feel full so that I stop eating. But when I eat fructose, none of that happens.

That's right.

So if I'm eating food with a lot of sugar, I'm likely to keep eating for longer than I would otherwise, even for reasons that have nothing to do with taste.

Exactly. And this has been shown a number of times in experiments with humans. For example, in one study,[7] researchers brought hungry people into a lab and split them into two groups: one group that got a meal with fructose in it and another group that got a different meal with the same number of calories but with the fructose replaced by glucose. Then they asked them how hungry they were after the meal.

And the group that got the fructose meal was hungrier than the group that got the glucose meal?

Right. And when the experiment was over, they gave everyone a choice between getting more food or getting paid and, as you might expect, the people in the fructose group were more likely to choose the food.

Right.

The researchers also monitored brain activity in both groups while they were eating. They saw that the glucose meal caused changes in the hypothalamus but the fructose meal had no effect.

Right, because fructose doesn't affect any of the signals that the hypothalamus is monitoring.

Exactly.

So, basically, one of the many reasons that sugar is a problem is that when my brain is keeping track of how many calories I've eaten, the fructose doesn't get counted properly.

Drinks

That's right. And the problem is much worse if the sugar is part of a drink, like soda.

Soda is just empty calories, right?

Actually, I think saying that soda is just empty calories is giving it too much credit. It suggests that soda is just energy without any other nutrients.

Oh, so the real empty calories are starches like white bread and pasta because they're just long strings of glucose.

Exactly. Soda is much worse than that. First of all, it has fructose, which is bad for all the reasons we just discussed. And second of all, it's a drink.

Why does that matter?

Because the calories in drinks don't get counted properly.[8] So if something is both a drink *and* high in fructose, it's barely going to register. So soda isn't just empty calories – soda is invisible calories.

Right. Wait, why don't the calories in drinks get counted properly?

For the same reason that the calories in fructose don't get counted properly: until recently, the calories in drinks didn't matter. I mean, until recently, there were no calories in drinks. There was only water.

What about milk?

Like I said earlier, adult humans only started drinking milk a few thousand years ago.

Right. OK, hold on, I get why fructose might not get counted like glucose or fat if, for example, the cells in my gut that release ghrelin don't have a detector for it. But are you saying that if I eat the same exact thing as either a liquid or a solid, it will get counted differently?

Yes, that's what I'm saying.

How can that matter? I mean, by the time it actually gets digested, it's all going to be a mush anyway, right? How can my body tell the difference?

Well, there are a few differences between how liquids and solids are digested: liquids are usually digested a bit faster, for example. But the problem is not that your body can tell the difference between liquids and solids, it's that your brain can.

OK, sure. But why does that matter?

Remember, your brain controls a lot of what happens in your gut. Like the way it tells your pancreas to start releasing insulin at your normal lunch time even before you start eating. It can also control your ghrelin and a lot of your other gut signals.[9]

Um, OK.

Let me tell you about a simple experiment.[10] Researchers took two groups of people and fed them exactly the same snack. The only difference was that one group got the snack in a box describing it as an "indulgent, decadent dessert," while the other group got the snack in a box describing it as a "guilt-free, healthy snack."

And?

And when the researchers monitored changes in ghrelin after the snack, they saw that ghrelin went down in the people who thought they were eating a dessert but not in the people who thought they were eating a healthy snack.

Even though they ate exactly the same thing?

Right. So while your ghrelin, insulin and other gut signals do, of course, reflect what you actually eat, they're also strongly influenced by what your brain thinks you're eating.

OK, I understand what you're saying, but that doesn't sound like a very good system. If my brain controls my gut signals based on what it thinks I'm eating and then monitors those same signals in order to know what I'm really eating, isn't that circular?

Sort of. There's definitely a trade-off involved. On the one hand, by guessing about what you're eating, your brain can prepare your gut to process all the food that's about to come in. For example, by the time any glucose starts coming into your blood, there will already be insulin there to tell your muscles to start using it. If your brain is right about what you're eating, it's going to make things a lot more efficient. On the other hand, if your brain is wrong, it can definitely cause problems. But it's only going to be wrong about processed foods. After millions of years of evolution in an environment with unprocessed foods, your brain is pretty familiar with them. So if you eat mostly unprocessed foods, this system is going to be helpful.

But it won't be helpful if I drink something like soda, because my brain just doesn't think of it as food?

That's right. Let me tell you about a few more experiments.[11]

Go ahead.

OK. In one experiment, researchers took two groups of people and fed them exactly the same food in either liquid or solid form.

So it had the same number of calories and all that?

Yes, it was literally the same food. Like the same number of apples either whole or juiced.

OK, and what happened?

Well, I'm sure you can guess by now. The group that got the solid food had bigger changes in their gut signals, like ghrelin, and they also reported feeling more full. But the important thing is that the researchers also monitored what the two groups ate over the next 24 hours and they found that the group that got the solid food ate hundreds fewer calories than the group that got the liquid food.

Oh, wow.

Yeah. This experiment has been repeated many times with different kinds of liquid and solid food.[12] Basically, if you replace a solid meal with a liquid one that has the same number of calories, you'll end up eating something like 10–20 per cent more over the next 24 hours.

And all because my brain just doesn't think of liquids as food.

Pretty much. But these effects can be complicated. For example, researchers did another version of the same experiment where they told one half of the liquid group that they were getting "juice" and the other half of the liquid group that they were getting "soup."

But they were actually getting the same exact liquid?

Right, they just called it juice or soup depending on which group they were talking to.

OK, and what happened?

Over the next 24 hours, the juice group ate an extra few hundred calories, the same way the original liquid group did. But the soup group didn't: they only ate as much as the original solid group.

What? Why? Just because we think of soup as a food, not a drink?

Well, that's really the only possible explanation.

OK, I think I get the point. Drinks are trouble because my brain doesn't think of them as food, so it doesn't count the calories in them properly. And sugary drinks, like soda, are double trouble because fructose also doesn't get counted properly.

That's right. And just to be clear, juice is no better than soda.

What do you mean?

I mean that fruit juice has pretty much the same number of calories and the same amount of sugar as soda.[13]

But juice is healthy, right?

Why?

Because, you know, it's juice.

Right.

No, I mean, juice has vitamins and stuff.

OK. If I took a vitamin pill and dropped it into a soda, would you consider that to be healthy?

No.

So why would juice be healthy, then?

Well, fruit is healthy, right?

Right.

So are you saying that fruit becomes unhealthy all of the sudden when it gets turned into a liquid?

That's exactly what I'm saying. Remember, one of the key factors that determines if something is healthy is whether or not it encourages overeating.

And juice encourages overeating because the calories in it don't get counted correctly.

Right.

But what if it's fresh juice without any added sugar? I get that it will still be a bit of a problem because it's a liquid but it won't be as bad as soda because it will have a lot less sugar, right?

Well, I told you before that a large coke from McDonald's has 50 grams of fructose.

Right. So how many grams of fructose would be in the same amount of apple juice?

50 grams.[14]

What? That's with no added sugar?

Right.

But I thought you said that fruit didn't actually have that much sugar in it.

It doesn't. To get that much juice, you need to use more than a dozen apples.[15] Are you ever going to eat that many apples?

No.

Well...

But at least juice has real sugar, rather than the fake stuff that's in soda.

What do you mean?

Isn't soda usually made with high-fructose corn syrup or something like that?

I suppose so. But why does that matter?

Well, isn't high-fructose corn syrup worse for you than regular sugar?

No. Why would it be? Oh, because it's "high-fructose?"

Yeah, for one thing.

Right. The name is a bit misleading. High-fructose corn syrup is actually not much higher in fructose than regular sugar: it's usually 55 per cent or 60 per cent fructose instead of 50 per cent.[16]

Oh. But at least real sugar is natural.

Regular sugar isn't any more or less natural than high-fructose corn syrup. In both cases, the sugar is extracted directly from plants. It's just a lot cheaper to extract the sugar from corn than it is from other plants. Sugar, high-fructose corn syrup, honey, molasses – they're all pretty much the same.

OK, fine. So juice is just soda with vitamins?

That's right.

But what about smoothies? Those are a lot thicker, so maybe my brain thinks of them as food. And smoothies have a lot more of the fiber and other stuff from the fruit, right?

Yeah, sure, a smoothie is probably a better choice than juice. But why not just eat the fruit?

OK, fine.

Good. Now, let's get back to sugar.

Hold on, can I ask one more question first?

Sure, go ahead.

What about alcohol?

Well, in terms of metabolism, alcohol is just like fructose.[17]

Right. I know that both are processed in my liver.

Right. But if you drink too much alcohol too fast, your liver won't be able to keep up and some of it will get processed in your brain.

Oh, I see. So that's why I'll end up drunk if I drink quickly but not if I drink slowly?

Right.

OK. But does an alcoholic drink have a lot of calories?

That depends on how much alcohol is in it. A weak drink like beer has about the same number of calories as soda or juice.[18]

What about wine?

Well, wine is usually about two or three times stronger than beer, so it has about two or three times as many calories.[19]

And I guess a really strong drink like vodka or gin has many more?

Right.[20]

OK. And do the calories in alcoholic drinks get counted properly?

Oh, no, alcoholic drinks are invisible calories just like soda or juice. There have been a lot of studies showing that people eat the same amount whether or not they have alcoholic drinks before or during a meal.[21]

And they don't make up for it by eating less later on?

No.

But I thought having one drink per day was supposed to be good for you?

Well, I wouldn't go that far. That idea is based on correlation studies that found that people who have one drink per day are less likely to have a heart attack or a stroke than people who don't drink at all.[22]

But that could be for a lot of reasons.

Right. Now, it may well be that one drink per day really is good for you. But there have never been any experimental studies on humans to really test that and the correlation studies are too poorly controlled to be convincing on their own.

But what about animal studies? Or studies of cells in a dish? I mean, alcohol is a big deal, so we must know a lot about it, right?

Oh, sure. It's clear that drinking a lot of alcohol is bad for you – that's obvious. Processing too much alcohol can damage your liver just like fructose. What isn't clear is whether drinking a little bit of alcohol is better for you than drinking no alcohol at all. There are reasons to believe that it might be – for example, small amounts of alcohol can decrease inflammation – but it's hard to be sure.[23]

Oh, I see. But if I want to have a drink, I'm probably better off having a beer than a soda.

I suppose. But in either case, you're going to be stuck with a few hundred extra calories that won't get counted properly. So if you don't *really* want the beer or the soda then you should just have water.

Right.

Good. Now, let's get back to sugar.

Hold on, while we're talking about drinks, I just want to ask one more question. What about coffee?

Coffee itself doesn't have any calories.[24] Neither does tea.

Oh, so does that mean that coffee has no effect on my metabolism or weight regulation systems? I drink like three or four cups per day, so I need to know if that's something to worry about.

Well, while coffee doesn't have any calories, it does have a lot of chemicals in it.

Like caffeine?

Right. But also many others. Some of those chemicals can have strong effects on their own. But when you drink them all together in the small amounts that are in a real cup of coffee, the overall effect on your metabolic and weight regulation systems seems to be neutral.[25]

OK, so I don't need to worry about drinking too much coffee, then?

I wouldn't. If anything, drinking coffee is probably good for you. Correlation studies suggest that you're less likely to have a heart attack or a stroke if you drink a few cups of coffee per day than if you drink none at all.[26] So, if you like coffee, keep drinking it.

OK, good. Sorry, we can get back to sugar now.

Addiction II

Good. So it's important to recognize all of the effects that sugar has on your body: it causes inflammation, it disrupts your gut bacteria, it damages your liver, it doesn't make you feel full. But, ultimately, the real problem is the effect that sugar has on your brain. It just tastes too good. How many times have you heard someone say, "Oh, I'm really trying to lose weight but I just can't stop eating these vegetables!"? It just doesn't happen.

Right. So it comes back to the addiction idea that we were talking about a while back.

Listen, the scientists who study addiction still argue about whether sugar, or food in general, is *really* addictive, and they're going to keep arguing about it because that's what scientists do. But what they're arguing about are the details of the different chemical reactions that take place in your brain when you take a drug or eat something tasty. If you're just a regular person who is interested in healthy eating, I'm not sure how much those details matter. What matters is whether tasty foods can cause us to *behave* like people who are addicted to a drug. Remember, there's no blood test or brain scan that can be used to diagnose addiction or dependence. The diagnosis is based solely on behavioral patterns.

Right. Sorry, but what's the difference between addiction and dependence?

Oh, actually, there is no difference anymore.[27] Now there is only one "substance use disorder." The diagnosis is based on a list of behaviors: the more of those behaviors you display, the stronger your disorder. Why don't I take you through the list and you can tell me whether or not you think each behavior can be caused by tasty foods?

OK, sure.

OK. First is "taking the substance in larger amounts or for longer than you intended to."

Well, sure, isn't that just overeating?

Kind of. If you went into a meal intending to stuff yourself, I guess that wouldn't count. It only counts if you end up eating more than you intended to when you started the meal.

OK, sure, that happens all the time.

Right. Next is "wanting to cut down or stop using the substance but not managing to."

OK, that's every failed diet.

Yeah, that's a clear one. How about "spending a lot of time getting, using or recovering from use of the substance?"

Hmm. I don't know about that one. People obviously do put a lot of time and effort into getting food but they need to do that in order to survive, right?

That's right. That's one of the main problems with trying compare food and drugs: you actually need food to survive. Now you don't actually need sugar, so you could, at least in theory, treat sugar as if it were a drug. But, of course, we usually eat sugar together with other foods that we do need, so looking at the effects of sugar on behavior separately from everything else really isn't possible.

Right.

OK, what about "having cravings and urges to use the substance?"

That's a tricky one too, right? I guess hunger is a craving for food but it's also a perfectly normal feeling.

Right, because, again, you need food to survive. But what about when you feel full and stop eating your main meal and then suddenly find room for dessert? It's hard to see how that could have anything to do with survival. But you're right, the distinction between normal hunger and unhealthy cravings for food is always going to be a bit blurry. What about "not managing to do what you should at work, home or school, because of substance use?"

I don't know, maybe. But that probably only applies to people who end up really obese and lose their ability to function normally.

You're right, that one probably only applies to people who really overdo it. But, depending on where you draw the line, between 5 per cent and 10 per cent of all Americans would be classified as "severely obese."[28] That's pretty similar to the number that would be classified as having drug use disorders.[29] OK, how about "continuing to use the substance, even when it causes problems in relationships?"

Oh, sure. If someone ends up unhealthy, that can be difficult for everyone in their life.

No doubt. Next is "giving up important social, occupational or recreational activities because of substance use."

Again, I think that one probably only applies in extreme cases.

OK, what about "using the substance again and again, even when it puts you in danger?"

Sure. Everyone knows that overeating is bad for their health but a lot of people continue to do it anyway.

Right. And "continuing to use the substance, even when you know you have a physical or psychological problem that could have been caused or made worse by the substance?"

Sure. But isn't that the same as the last one?

Yeah, more or less. "Needing more of the substance to get the effect you want?"

That's tolerance, right? I don't know. Does that happen?

Well, this is another tricky one. I mean, bigger people need more calories to maintain their weight, so it makes sense that as you continue to overeat and gain weight, you will need to eat more to feel full. But, beyond that, it does seem that the same tasty foods can bring you less and less pleasure over time.[30] The last one is "development of withdrawal symptoms, which can be relieved by taking more of the substance."

Well, that's just hunger, right? So that's another tricky one.

Right. OK, so if we ignore the behaviors that might be caused by normal hunger, we're left with five behaviors that are common in many people who are overweight. That's enough to qualify as a "moderate" use disorder. And if we add in the two that we said probably only apply in extreme cases, we're up to seven, which qualifies as a "severe" disorder. Now, if you want to get technical like the scientists and start comparing the changes happening inside your brain when you take drugs or eat tasty food, you'll find some differences. But you'll also find a lot of similarities. Do you remember what we said about how your pleasure system works?

Oh, well... actually, no, I don't, I'm sorry.

That's OK, it's been a while since we talked about it. Let me remind you. When you eat something tasty, cells in your brain release opioids and cannabinoids, which are the two pleasure chemicals.

Right, so tasty food causes my brain to release its own heroin and marijuana.

Right. And once your brain learns that a certain food tastes good, it will start to release the craving chemical, dopamine, whenever you see it.

Or anything that reminds me of it.

Right. And the dopamine will tell other parts of your brain to do whatever they need to do to get the food.

OK, I remember now. And the only way I can resist these cravings is if my self-control system cancels the orders sent by the dopamine.

Right. Your self-control system can shut down the brain cells that would have carried out the order sent by the dopamine.

Right. My self-control system can inhibit the behavior but not the craving.

Exactly, so if the cravings are too strong or you have them too often, your self-control will eventually break down.

OK, got it.

Good. So what do you think happens when you become addicted to something?

Well, I guess my cravings for it keep getting stronger and stronger and become harder and harder to satisfy.

Right. Now, normally, when you're hungry and you start eating a food that you haven't eaten in a while, your brain will release a lot of dopamine at first but it will gradually release less and less as you keep eating it.

Why, because I'll start getting full?

Oh, yes, if you're just talking about one meal. But I'm talking about what happens after many meals over several days. If you eat the same thing day after day, your brain will release less and less dopamine each time.

Why?

Well, from an evolutionary perspective, this makes sense because it encourages you to eat a mix of different foods. That way, you're sure to get all of the different nutrients that you need.

Oh, OK, sure.

But with drugs, this doesn't happen. If you take a drug regularly, your brain will release more and more dopamine each time and your craving for it will just keep getting stronger.[31]

Right.

Now, here's the thing: that also happens with sugar.[32]

Really?

Really. I mean, this kind of thing is hard to measure directly in humans but it's very clear in animals. Researchers have been doing experiments to test the effects of drugs on animals for a long time and they see all of the behaviors that you would expect to see in addicted humans: bingeing, craving, tolerance, withdrawal. Now, they've started doing the same experiments with sugar and they see a lot of the same things.[33]

Wow.

I really don't want to get into this too deeply but let me just tell you about one study.[34]

Go ahead.

OK. So researchers did a series of experiments in which they took rats and put them into a box with two levers. At the beginning of each day, the rats were allowed to push each lever twice to see what happened. After those initial presses, they were allowed eight more presses of whichever lever they wanted. After those eight presses, they were done for the day.

OK...

For one group of rats, they used a box where one lever gave them cocaine but the other lever did nothing. What do you think happened?

I guess the rats used their initial presses to figure out which lever gave them the cocaine and they used all of their other eight presses on that one?

That's right. For a second group of rats, they used a different box where one lever gave them sugar but the other lever did nothing.

OK. And I guess those rats figured out which lever gave them the sugar and they used all of their eight presses on that one?

Right. Nothing too surprising so far. But now, for a third group of rats, they used a different box where one lever gave them sugar and the other lever gave them cocaine.

Oh, don't tell me they chose the sugar!

Almost every time.

C'mon.

I'm serious.

OK, was it a huge dose of sugar and a tiny dose of cocaine?

No, they tried it with a lot of different doses and always got the same results. But, wait, there's more. Next, they took the rats that had been in the cocaine-only box for a few weeks and started putting them in the cocaine-and-sugar box.

Don't tell me they started choosing the sugar over the cocaine?

Almost every one of them.

Stop it.

I know. It's hard to believe but the results were very consistent.

So you're saying that sugar is more addictive than cocaine?

I don't know. I'm not saying anything. I only brought it up just to give you some idea about the kinds of experiments that are being done. Whether or not sugar or other foods are technically addictive doesn't matter.

So what does matter?

10
Diets

Knowledge

What matters is that many, many people are unhealthy and unhappy because they are overweight and they want to stop overeating but they can't seem to manage it.

You're right that there are a lot of people who want to stop overeating and can't. But it's not as if they're not trying. Listen, I'm not trying to be rude, I really appreciate the time you've taken to tell me all of this. But, in the end, what you're telling me is that unprocessed foods are healthy and processed foods are not. Don't most people kind of know that already? I mean, you've made the problem very clear: people eat too many processed foods. But you haven't really offered a solution.

Well, now, hold on, I think your overall point is a fair one and I'll come back to it. But there are a couple things I'd like to clarify. First of all, I think there are actually a lot of people who don't think in terms of processed and unprocessed and might not have the right idea about which foods are healthy and which aren't. For example, I think there are a lot of people who would think that they were making a healthy choice by buying something that said "low fat" on the front and they wouldn't necessarily look at the back to see if it had a lot of sugar in it. I mean, a few minutes ago, you thought that fruit juice was healthy, didn't you?

Maybe.

Right. So I think there are still a lot of misunderstandings about which foods are healthy and which aren't. And, also, I do think that there is a difference between just knowing whether a food is healthy

or unhealthy and really understanding *why* it's healthy or unhealthy. I think that if you really understand the details of why processed foods are unhealthy, it's going to be easier to avoid them.

Why?

Well, let's say it's time for an afternoon snack and you have to choose between a piece of cake and a piece of fruit. You might say to yourself, "Oh, that cake looks good but it's unhealthy, so I should eat the fruit instead."

Right.

The problem is that if you don't understand the details of exactly why cake is unhealthy, you might be able to talk yourself into the cake by saying something like "Wait, am I really sure that cake is unhealthy? It seems like the experts change their minds every week about which foods are healthy and which foods aren't. Am I depriving myself for no good reason?"

Right.

But since you do understand the details of exactly why cake is unhealthy, that kind of argument isn't going to work. You can respond with "What are you talking about? The real experts aren't changing their minds about anything. The consensus among scientists about which foods are healthy or unhealthy, and why, hasn't changed for years. The reasons why cake is unhealthy are perfectly clear. The biggest problem is that cake has a lot of sugar in it. Sugar will increase my inflammation, disrupt my gut bacteria, damage my liver and encourage me to overeat because it tastes so good and the calories in it aren't counted properly. And the fact that cake doesn't have any fiber doesn't help either. Because cake doesn't have any fiber, it doesn't feed the gut bacteria that feed my intestinal wall cells, it's more calorie dense and the glucose in it gets digested quickly and causes an insulin overshoot. The extra insulin will cause my blood glucose to drop below normal and prevent my fat cells from releasing fat. And my brain will respond to the low blood glucose and fat by making me feel of hungry or tired, which will just encourage me to eat even more and be less active. So, yeah, I'm sure that cake is unhealthy."

OK, I see your point. If I understand the details of why processed foods are unhealthy, it's going to be hard for me to ignore those details and make the decision to eat processed foods anyway.

Well, maybe not hard but at least hard*er*. I mean, even if you know all the details and really believe that processed foods are unhealthy, resisting them might still be a struggle. Which brings us back to your original point: there are many people who know perfectly well which foods are healthy and unhealthy and why but still end up overweight.

Right. So what's the solution? What kind of diet actually works?

Diets

Well, that's the billion dollar question, isn't it? I do think there is an answer but it's unlikely to be any kind of traditional diet – you know, a plan that prescribes eating specific foods in specific amounts. I think those kinds of plans are really missing the point.

What do you mean?

First of all, there really isn't any strong evidence suggesting that any particular foods are better or worse for you than others.

Wait, what? What have we been talking about this whole time? Aren't foods that cause inflammation, disrupt gut bacteria or promote overeating worse than foods that don't?

Oh, of course. Wait, hold on, I'm assuming that we're only talking about unprocessed foods. I mean, if you're still not convinced that processed foods are generally unhealthy then I give up.

No, sure, that's fine. I was just confused.

OK, so processed foods are out. What I'm saying is that, beyond that, it's hard to make the case for any one particular mix of unprocessed foods over any other.[1] Maybe being a vegetarian is a little better than going paleo or maybe the Mediterranean diet is a little better than the South Beach diet...

Wait, what's the South Beach diet again?

I don't know; forget it. The point is that it's impossible to say that any one of those diets is that much better than any other. And there's really no reason to think that any one particular mix of unprocessed foods *should* be that much better than any other. We're generalists, not specialists.

What do you mean?

Our ancestors had very little control over the particular mix of foods they ate; they had no choice but to eat whatever they could find. So we evolved to be able to stay healthy while eating a range of different foods, not to thrive on any one particular mix. Anyway, you can always find one study that favors a particular mix of foods over others if you want to. But if you really consider all of the available evidence, they all look about the same in the end.

So none of them work?

No, all of them work! Or at least all of them *can* work, because they all focus on unprocessed foods. If you're worried about inflammation, gut bacteria and overeating, then the important thing to do is to cut out processed foods. If you can do that – and I mean *really* do it – then you're going to be fine. Any diet that is a mix of all the different kinds of unprocessed foods – vegetables, fruits, meats, poultry, fish, whole grains, nuts and dairy – is going to work if you can stick to it.

Wait, aren't dairy products processed?

Oh, that's a good question. Technically, yes. Unless you're drinking milk straight from the cow, any dairy products that you buy will have been processed. But most dairy processing involves either removing or adding bacteria, both of which are fine. Milk is usually heated to kill bacteria and cheese and yogurt usually have bacteria added to them.

Oh, do the bacteria that are added to cheese and yogurt interact with gut bacteria?

Probably,[2] but those interactions haven't really been studied in detail yet, so it's hard to say for sure. If anything, it seems like the bacteria added to cheese and yogurt are helpful, not harmful, so that's not the kind of processing you need to worry about.[3] What you need to worry about are all of the other additives that you would find in any processed food.

Like preservatives or sugar?

Right. But dairy products without additives aren't that hard to find. Any big grocery store will usually have a few choices. And if you can get to a farmer's market or something like that, it'll really be no problem.

Personalized advice

OK, hold on. So you're saying that it doesn't matter whether my diet is high in fat and low in carbs or vice versa?

Well, most of your cells are happy to use either glucose or fat for energy, right? What I'm saying is that when your metabolic systems are working properly, your body is going to be able to adapt to whatever you eat – within reason, of course.[4] If you eat a lot of glucose, your pancreas will release a lot of insulin and your cells will use a lot of glucose for energy. If you eat a lot of fat, your pancreas will release very little insulin and your cells will use a lot of fat for energy. There have been a lot of experimental studies where humans are put on diets that are high in fat and low in carbs or vice versa and, on average, the results are usually pretty similar.[5] Now, it may well be that *you* would be better off eating more fat than carbs or vice versa, but we can never really know that.

Why not?

How could we? I mean, if we had thousands of identical copies of you and a few decades to run experiments on them, we might be able to figure out your ideal diet but, obviously, that's not going to happen.

But can't I just get my genes scanned? Or get a blood test?

That's not going to help. Unfortunately, at the moment, it's not really possible to get personalized dietary advice that is both detailed and accurate. Let me give you a simple example.[6] Dietary advice for people with diabetes usually has one primary goal: to keep blood glucose levels as low as possible. So the general advice would be to avoid foods with a lot of glucose that is easily digested.

Right. So that means avoiding foods with a high glycemic index, right?

Sort of. It's really glycemic load, not glycemic index, that's important.

What's the difference?

Glycemic index tells you how easily the glucose in a food is digested but it doesn't tell you how much glucose is actually in the food. Glycemic load tells you both.

Oh, I see. So something can have a high glycemic index but, if it doesn't actually have much glucose in it, then it doesn't really matter?

Right. Carrots, for example, have a high glycemic index but a low glycemic load.[7] So if you eat a carrot, the glucose from it will go straight into your blood but, since carrots don't actually have that much glucose in them, it doesn't really matter. Something like pasta, on the other hand, that has a lot of easily digestible glucose will have both a high glycemic index and a high glycemic load.[8]

OK, so it's really the glycemic load that matters.

Right. So the general advice given to people with diabetes is to avoid foods with a high glycemic load. And this, of course, is perfectly good advice that is generally effective for most people. However, there are also huge differences between people: the same food can make one person's blood glucose jump but have almost no effect on someone else.

Why?

Well, it could be for a lot of reasons. Maybe it has to do with the exact details of how and where their inflammation is interfering with their insulin. Or maybe one person's gut bacteria are really helpful for digesting a certain kind of starch and the other person's aren't. The problem is that many of the relevant details are impossible to measure, at least with current technology. And, even if we could measure them, we still don't know enough to be able to use them to predict how a particular food is going to change a particular person's blood glucose.

So giving diabetic people more personalized eating advice doesn't help?

Not really. They just have to learn by trial and error. Now, don't get me wrong, when we finally do have the technology and knowledge to give people personalized eating advice that is accurate, it's going to be incredibly useful. I fantasize about having a smart toilet that knows all about me and can analyze my urine and feces and tell me what I should be eating.

Don't we all...

Unfortunately, we're just not there yet. So all you can really do is just eat a reasonable mix of unprocessed foods and see what happens.

Salt

OK. But what about saturated fats and red meat? Wouldn't we all be better off if we cut those out? The evidence that they might cause inflammation and disrupt gut bacteria seemed strong enough.

You're right, the animal studies have certainly made it very clear how saturated fats and red meat can cause inflammation and disrupt gut bacteria. And the human studies do suggest that a diet that is very high in either or both might be harmful. So, OK, I guess you're right, going easy on the saturated fats and red meat is probably a good idea. But there are two reasons why you might not want to cut them out altogether. First of all, if you do, you're going to have to put a lot more thought into what you eat.

What do you mean?

We've spent a lot of time talking about different kinds of carbs and fats but there are a lot of other things in food that we haven't discussed at all.

Right, like protein or vitamins and minerals.

Right. Those things are incredibly important,[9] but as long as you eat a reasonable mix of unprocessed foods, you'll get everything you need and you won't have to think about them.

What about salt? I know it's important but we haven't talked about it at all yet.

You're right, salt is important. But it's another thing you don't have to think about as long as you eat mostly unprocessed foods. It's only the large amounts of salt that are added to processed foods that can become a problem.[10]

But why would too much salt ever be a problem? Salt doesn't have any calories, right? Oh, wait, it has something to do with blood pressure, doesn't it?

That's right. Salt doesn't have any calories, so you can't use it for energy. But it's one of the key chemicals in your body, like oxygen or water, and keeping the right amount of it in your blood is extremely important.[11] So one of the main jobs of your kidneys is to filter any extra salt out of your blood and into your urine.

But what does that have to do with blood pressure?

Blood pressure is a measure of how hard your heart is pushing your blood through your body. The harder your blood is pushed through your kidneys, the more salt they will filter out.

Oh, OK. So if I eat too much salt, my blood pressure will increase to help my kidneys get rid of the extra salt?

That's right. But that only happens as a last resort. When your kidneys are working properly, they'll actually simply adjust themselves to filter out more or less salt as needed and your blood pressure won't change. But if you start gaining weight and fat starts building up around your kidneys, they'll eventually stop working properly.[12] When that happens, then your blood pressure will increase because that will be the only way to get extra salt out.

I see. And why is high blood pressure a problem? It's supposed to make a heart attack or a stroke more likely, right?

That's right.[13] If you have high blood pressure, it means that your heart is always pushing hard.

And if it has to push too hard for too long, it eventually burns out?

Right, that's heart failure.[14] But high blood pressure isn't only bad for your heart, it's also bad for your blood vessels. The high pressure can damage the walls of your blood vessels and make it easier for fat packages to get stuck and for plaques to build up.[15]

Oh, OK. So that's why having high blood pressure makes a heart attack or a stroke more likely?

Right.

OK, got it. But I don't need to worry about any of this as long as my kidneys are working properly. So as long as I'm lean and healthy, I don't need to think about how much salt I eat?

Not really. I mean, I guess it's possible to overdo it if you eat a lot of processed foods,[16] but otherwise the amount of salt in your blood will stay pretty much the same no matter what you eat.[17]

OK. But if I'm overweight and my kidneys aren't working properly, I need to be more careful.

Exactly.[18] But all you would have to do is switch from eating processed foods to eating unprocessed foods, which, if you're overweight, is something you should be doing anyway.

OK, so as long as I stick to mostly unprocessed foods, I'll get enough of all the vitamins and minerals and everything else that I need and I'll avoid getting too much of anything that might be harmful.

That's right.

Supplements and superfoods

And are there any particular vitamins or minerals that I should really try to get a lot of?

How, with supplements? No. As long as you're eating a reasonable mix of unprocessed foods, you'll get all the vitamins and minerals you need and getting more of them isn't going to help. In fact, if anything, it's going to hurt: the huge amounts of vitamins and minerals that you get from supplements can cause problems.[19]

So you wouldn't even take a multi-vitamin?

No. Why would I? There is no evidence that multi-vitamins or any other supplements are helpful.[20] Even fish fats, which we know have the potential to be helpful, don't seem to have much of an effect when you take them as supplements.[21]

But how can fish fats be good for me when I eat them in fish but not when I take them as supplements?

Well, hold on. I never said that there was any direct evidence that fish fats are good for you when you eat them in fish. What I said was that people who eat a lot of fish fats are healthier than people who don't.[22] Now, that might be because of the fish fats – they certainly had strong effects in the animal studies that we discussed. But there's another possibility that's much simpler. If you're eating more fish, that means that you're eating less of something else and that something else might be processed foods.

So people who eat a lot of fish fats might be healthier simply because they eat fewer processed foods?

Maybe. When you eat fish, not only are you eating something that might be good for you, you're also *not* eating something that might be bad for you. But if you just take fish fat supplements without changing what you eat otherwise, that's not the case.

Right.

Listen, even if researchers do eventually find out that particular foods or supplements really are good for you, they're not going to be *that* good for you. Any direct benefits that you can get from eating particular foods are going to be tiny compared to the damage that you can do by overeating processed foods. This is why I think it's

misleading to talk about "healthy foods" versus "unhealthy foods." Those terms suggest that there is some sort of symmetry, which is just not the case.

What do you mean?

I mean that you can harm yourself much more by eating a lot of "unhealthy foods" than you can help yourself by eating a lot of "healthy foods."

Right. I guess you can't undo the effects of eating fast food for lunch everyday just by eating salads for dinner.

Right. The best thing about "healthy foods" is really just that they're not "unhealthy foods." So instead of talking about "healthy foods" versus "unhealthy foods," it would be better to just talk about "foods" versus "unhealthy foods."

So I guess you're not into "superfoods" then?[23]

Oh, sure I am. Blueberries, spinach, almonds – I love all of those things and I eat them all the time. But I don't believe that the chemicals in them are going to somehow keep me lean and healthy even if I overeat processed foods the rest of the time.

Diets II

OK, OK. So I should just generally stick to unprocessed foods and not overthink it.

That's right. Unless you decide to start cutting out whole categories of food – that's a different story. For example, you suggested earlier that we might be better off if we cut out saturated fats because they can increase inflammation and disrupt gut bacteria.

Right. But you said there were two reasons why that might not be a good idea.

Right. First of all, you'd have to put a lot more thought into what you ate. Cutting out saturated fats would basically mean cutting out meat and dairy. But if you did that, there would be a lot of important things that you might not get enough of, like calcium, iodine, iron or zinc. If your diet includes meat and dairy, then you're going to get plenty of those things. But if it doesn't, then you have to be careful about choosing the particular mix of foods that you eat. You can still get everything you need but it's going to require some thought.[24]

I see.

So if you feel really strongly that cutting out meat and dairy is the right thing to do for ethical or environmental reasons, then go for it. But if you're worried only about your health, then I think you're better off including them in your diet. The risks associated with having some – not a lot but some – saturated fats and red meats in your diet appear to be minimal,[25] and the benefit of not having to think so much about what you eat is, at least for me, huge. I mean, eating only unprocessed foods is enough of an effort as it is; do you really want to be worrying, "Oh, did I get enough zinc this week?" From a health perspective, I don't think it's worth the hassle.

Right.

But there's another really good reason to include meat and dairy in your diet: you like them. If you want to have any hope of sticking to a diet, you have to enjoy it. You want to know what kind of diet actually works? One that you can actually stick to.[26] We can agree now that if you want to be lean and healthy, you need to eat a mix of unprocessed foods, right?

Right.

Good. So that also means that, if you want to be lean and healthy, you need to avoid eating processed foods, right?

Right, and I guess that's the really hard part.

Of course it is! Processed foods are convenient and cheap and they taste really, really good. Remember, eating, just like all behavior, is a battle between your pleasure system and your self-control system. If you have to use your self-control system to overrule your pleasure system every time you make a decision about eating, you're eventually going to break down and end up back on the processed foods. If you want to have any hope of sticking to a diet, you have to enjoy it. Forget about which mix of unprocessed foods is the healthiest. Like I said, there's no real evidence to favor any one particular mix anyway. The important thing is to find the mix of unprocessed foods that you enjoy the most because that's the one you're most likely to be able to stick to.

OK, listen, I'm fine with the idea that any reasonable mix of unprocessed food is going to be healthy. But the suggestion that everyone is going to magically be able to resist processed foods just by finding their favorite mix of unprocessed foods sounds pretty naïve. I mean, what about people who try all kinds of different diets but can't stick to any of them? Are you just saying they haven't found the right one? I think resisting processed foods is a lot harder than you're making it out to be. Do you really not eat *any* processed foods?

Of course I do! Haven't you detected a clear personal undertone in all of our discussions of sugar addiction? I tried giving up sugar once – I didn't even make it through the afternoon.

Are you serious? So you still haven't solved the problem?

Hold on, I'm not saying that you need to eat *only* unprocessed foods. I'm saying that you need to eat *mostly* unprocessed foods. If you wanted to be as healthy as possible, you might need to exclude processed foods altogether. But you don't need to be as healthy as possible – you just need to be healthy. Most people can eat a terrible diet that is mostly processed foods and still only gain a few pounds per year.

But if you do that for too long, you're going to end up obese.

Of course. I'm not suggesting that anyone should eat mostly processed foods. I'm simply saying that your diet doesn't need to be perfect. The problem with trying to eat a perfect diet is that you probably won't enjoy it enough to stick to it. Now, that would be fine if you eventually settled on a diet that was less than perfect but still mostly unprocessed foods. But that's not what happens, right? Most people who fail to stick to a perfect diet end up all the way back at an unhealthy diet that is mostly processed foods.

OK, sure, a perfect diet probably isn't going to work. But there are plenty of people who have tried more realistic diets that include some processed foods and haven't been able to stick to those either.

You're right. Recognizing that your diet doesn't need to be perfect is just the first step. If you want to avoid sliding back into an unhealthy diet, you also need to establish a regular eating routine and make a lot of changes to your environment.

Oh, c'mon. Are you trying to tell me that eating breakfast at the same time every morning with the right music in the background is going to solve all of my problems?

Of course not. There's never going to be any one change that will solve all of your problems. But a lot of small changes together can make a big difference. And, actually, eating all of your meals at the same time each day is a great place to start. Meal timing is something that scientists have been studying a lot but, for whatever reason, hasn't got a lot of media attention.[27]

But why does it matter *when* you eat? Isn't it *what* you eat that's important?

What you eat is extremely important, of course, and we've established that what you eat should be mostly a mix of unprocessed foods. But if you try just telling yourself "OK, from now on, I'm going to eat mostly a mix of unprocessed foods," you're probably not going to stick to it. So you should do whatever else you can to give yourself every advantage, right?

Sure. But is eating at the right times really going to help?

Absolutely.

But why?

11
Daily rhythms and meal timing

Daily rhythms

When you eat is important for several reasons. The first has to do with the daily rhythms in your body and brain.[1] If you eat at the right times, you'll reinforce your daily rhythms and they will work to your advantage. If you eat at the wrong times, you'll disrupt your daily rhythms and you'll be in trouble. The bottom line is that if you do most of your eating during the day when it's light outside, you'll be leaner and healthier than if you eat the same exact food at random times throughout the day and night.

Oh, c'mon. How is that possible? I'm sorry, but if you want me to believe any of this you're going to have to give me a lot more detail. First of all, what are these daily rhythms that you're talking about?

All of the cells in your body have daily rhythms: they do more of some things during the day and more of other things at night.

Why?

For efficiency. Our ancestors had no electricity, so they were forced to stick to a pretty regular schedule: they would seek and eat food during the day and they would rest and sleep at night.

Sure.

So if you know that you're going to stick to a schedule like that, there's no point in, for example, wasting energy preparing your intestinal wall cells for incoming food in the middle of the night, right?

I guess not.

Nor is there any point in trying to do maintenance work inside those cells during the day when incoming food is likely to keep getting in the way. It's better to leave the maintenance until it can be done without interruption.

Right, like the way office buildings are cleaned overnight rather than during the day when all of the workers are there.

Right. So our ancestors evolved daily rhythms to organize the activity in their cells around their normal schedule. During the day, cells prepare for activity in general and also for whatever it is they do during eating: intestinal wall cells get ready to digest food, pancreas cells get ready to release insulin, liver cells get ready to store glucose and so on. At night, cells clean up waste and repair damaged parts and prepare for whatever it is that they do during sleep.

OK, that makes sense. But how do my cells know whether it's day or night?

There's a tiny part of your brain – your brain clock – that sends them messages.[2]

How?

The usual ways. Your brain clock can use hormones to send indirect chemical messages or it can use nerves to send direct electrical messages.

And how does my brain clock know what time it is?

It mostly just keeps track of light and dark.

Fine.

Good. So you can imagine that these daily rhythms gave our ancestors a big advantage: because they were more efficient, they could survive on less food.

Right, I'm with you.

OK. But, of course, nowadays, we don't limit our eating to the daylight hours.

Right, but why is that a problem? I mean, food isn't scarce anymore, so we can afford to be a little less efficient, can't we?

Right. But it's not just about energy efficiency. When you eat at night, you catch your cells off guard and force them to process and store glucose and fat when they're unprepared.

Why does that matter?

Well, remember, overwhelming your cells with glucose or fat is one of the surest ways to increase inflammation.

Right, that's the backlog-driven inflammation that we talked about: if my immune cells notice a build-up of waste and half-processed glucose and fat, they'll take action.

Right. And if your cells are unprepared, they're going to be more easily overwhelmed.

I see.

And if you eat late at night and then again early in the morning, you won't be giving your cells a long enough break to get their maintenance done. So they might end up with a build-up of junk or damage, which will also increase inflammation.

Right.

Now, as with most things, eating at night is no big deal if you do it every once in a while. But if you do it all the time, your cells will never have time to do their maintenance and, eventually, your daily rhythms will break down.

Why?

Because if your brain clock and your behavior are always out of sync, your cells will end up confused. On the one hand, when it's dark outside, your brain clock will be telling them that they should be doing their maintenance and preparing for what they normally do at night. But, on the other hand, if you keep eating at night, you'll keep forcing your cells to do the things they normally do during the day.

OK, so if my brain clock is telling my cells to do one thing but my behavior is forcing them to do another, my daily rhythms will break down.

Right. It's like when two people try to push a child on a swing: it'll only work if they both push at the same time. Your brain clock is always going to push your cells one way during the day and the other way at night. If you want your daily rhythms to stay strong, you need to make sure that your behavior is always pushing your cells the same way as your brain clock.

OK, I understand why catching my cells off guard and not giving them time to do their maintenance might be a problem. But why is it a problem if my daily rhythms break down? I mean, shouldn't that actually help? If my cells just start doing a bit of everything all the time then maybe they'll be less unprepared when I eat at night. Or maybe they'll be able to get a little maintenance done during the day. It seems like having no rhythms at all would be better than having rhythms that are out of sync with my behavior.

Right. Unfortunately, your cells don't just start doing a bit of everything all the time when your daily rhythms break down. In fact, what happens is that instead of doing more or less of certain things at certain times, your cells just start doing more or less of certain things *all of the time.*[3] **For example, when your daily rhythms are working, your liver will make and release a large amount of glucose at night but only a small amount during the day. But when your rhythms break down, your liver doesn't just release a medium amount of glucose all the time, it releases a large amount of glucose all the time, which means that it will release more glucose overall.**

I see.

And the same kind of thing happens in all of your cells: when your daily rhythms break down, your pancreas cells will release more insulin overall, your fat cells will release less leptin overall, the cells in your gut will release less ghrelin overall. I could go on and on but I'm sure you get the point.

Daily rhythms II

OK, so, basically, if my daily rhythms break down, everything goes haywire.

Yeah, pretty much.

OK, I can see why that would be a problem, but does it really happen?

Oh, definitely. Should I tell you about some experiments?

Yes, please.

OK, let's start with some animal experiments.[4] In the first one, researchers split mice into two groups and overfed both groups with food that had a lot of sugar and fat. The only difference was that one group could access the food anytime they wanted but the other group could only access it during the half of the day that they were normally active.

So the half-day mice were forced to keep their behavior in sync with their brain clock but the all-day mice weren't?

Exactly. The all-day mice just ate at random times throughout the day and night.

OK, so the daily rhythms broke down in the all-day mice but not in the half-day mice?

Right.

And I guess you're going to tell me that the all-day mice gained weight and the half-day mice didn't?

That's right. And the all-day mice developed all of the usual problems that go along with being overweight – inflammation, insulin resistance, liver damage – but the half-day mice didn't. In fact, the half-day mice were just as healthy as mice would normally be on their natural diet.

But isn't that just because the all-day mice ate more than the half-day mice?

No, that's the thing, they didn't. Both groups of mice ate the same amount of food overall. The only difference was that the all-day mice spread their eating throughout the day and night.

OK, so were the all-day mice less active? Did they just sit around between meals?

Nope. Both groups of mice were equally active.

So the half-day mice just magically burned more calories than the all-day mice?

Well, there's really nothing magical about it. The metabolic and weight regulation systems in the all-day mice weren't working properly at all: their livers were constantly making glucose, their fat cells were constantly storing fat rather than releasing it and so on.

But if two mice eat the same amount of food and do the same amount of activity, then shouldn't they be the same weight?

No! We talked about how you can burn a different number of calories doing the same amount of activity depending on whether your cells are trying to save energy or trying to waste it by creating heat.

Oh, right, I remember. So the half-day mice burned off a lot of extra calories by wasting energy and the all-day mice didn't?

Right.

Wow, OK. I know you said that wasting energy was a big deal but I didn't realize it was *that* big of a deal. I mean, I didn't realize it could make the difference between being overweight or not.

Oh, sure.

Are there mutant mice that are unable to waste energy by creating heat?

Yes, and they gain much more weight when they're overfed than normal mice.[5] In fact, they even become obese on a normal diet.

Really? And that's not because they eat more or are less active than normal mice?

Nope. It's just because their cells are unable to waste energy.

That's pretty amazing.

I agree.

Gut bacteria rhythms

OK, and the all-day mice had all of these problems just because the daily rhythms in their cells were disrupted?

Right. And the daily rhythms in their gut bacteria as well, of course.

Right. Wait, what? Gut bacteria also have daily rhythms?

Sure. Well, the individual bacteria themselves don't, of course, because they never live for a whole day. But the changes in the particular mix of bacteria in your gut will have a daily rhythm that reflects your behavior.[6] For example, if you eat mostly during the day, then bacteria that live off food or chemicals related to digestion will have a better chance of surviving and reproducing during the day than they will at night.

But how does that affect me?

The daily rhythms in your bacteria are important for reinforcing the daily rhythms in some of the cells that are close to your gut. When researchers did experiments comparing the daily rhythms in normal mice with the daily rhythms in bacteria-free mice or mice that were on antibiotics, they saw that the mice without gut bacteria had much

weaker rhythms in their intestinal wall cells, their gut immune cells and even in their livers.[7]

Sorry, hold on. I don't really see how the rhythms in my gut bacteria can influence the rhythms in my other cells?

The rhythms in your "other cells?" I like that – it sounds like you're starting to think of your gut bacteria as a part of you! Anyway, it's not so different from the way that eating influences your daily rhythms. The same way your cells normally expect to receive incoming glucose and fat at certain times, they also expect to receive things from your bacteria at certain times.

Like what?

Like the fat that your gut bacteria make when they digest fiber. When those fiber fats stop coming, it disrupts your daily rhythms.

OK, so it's not the bacteria themselves, it's just the things that they make?

It's both. In the same experiments, the researchers gave the mice that were on antibiotics injections of fiber fats at the same time each day and they saw that some of the daily rhythms in their livers returned but others didn't. So the rhythms that didn't return after the fiber fat injections were probably dependent directly on the bacteria themselves.

But why?

Remember, your gut immune cells are constantly patrolling your intestinal walls and they're used to detecting more of some bacteria during the day and more of other bacteria at night. If you start eating at random times throughout the day and night and disrupt the rhythms in your gut bacteria, your gut immune cells will end up making the wrong detectors and chemicals at the wrong times. And you can imagine how that can lead to a leaky gut with bacteria getting into your blood, increased inflammation and so on.

OK, I get it. But does this kind of thing actually happen in humans?

Meal timing

Well, there are a lot of correlation studies that suggest that behaviors that are out of sync with your brain clock cause problems.

People who work the night shift, for example, are much more likely than other people to be overweight or have diabetes, heart attacks or strokes.[8] And people who are obese and diabetic generally have weaker daily rhythms than people who are lean and healthy.[9]

But those correlations could have a lot of different causes, right? Have there been any experimental studies?

There have and the results seem to point in the same direction as the correlation studies. There have been a few studies where people were brought into a lab for a week or so and forced to eat at different times throughout the day and night.[10] Studies like that are always too short to tell us anything about long-term effects but they're helpful for trying to understand how the problems start. For example, one study found that even after just a few days of eating at night, your fat cells will release a lot less leptin overall.

But the basic idea is that doing most of your eating during the day is better than eating at random times throughout the day and night, right?

Right.

So why don't researchers just get a group of overweight people to start eating only during the day for a few months to see if that helps them lose weight? Even if it's not well-controlled, they might still see something, right?

Right. That's a good idea and it has been done.[11]

Oh. And?

It works.

Great! So what exactly did they do?

Just what you suggested. Researchers got a group of overweight people and told them to keep eating whatever they wanted to, and as much as they wanted to, but only during the day. Everyone chose exactly when they wanted to eat but most people stuck to the period between 9am and 8pm.

Was the study done in a lab?

No.

OK, so how did the researchers know if the people really followed the instructions?

They gave them a smartphone app and told them to take a photo of every meal and snack they ate. The app sent the photos to the researchers automatically, so they were able to keep track of what, when and how much everyone ate.

But surely the people didn't photograph everything.

No, I'm sure they didn't. That's the problem with doing a long-term study in the real world instead of a lab. But the photos are probably better than asking people to write everything down.

OK, so they lost weight?

Right. After 16 weeks, they lost an average of seven pounds.

Hey, that's pretty good!

It is. And what's even better is that the people in the study actually liked doing most of their eating during the day. In fact, they all voluntarily agreed to keep it up. And when the researchers checked them again after a year, they hadn't regained any of the weight.

Wow.

Yeah. But there was one problem.

What?

Well, it's not really a problem, it's just a complication: the people in the study didn't just change *when* they ate, they also changed *how much* they ate. They actually ate an average of 20 per cent less overall.

So they ate less without being told to?

Right.

OK, so that's different from the study with the all-day and half-day mice, right? The half-day mice just ate the same amount of food in less time. These people actually ate less food in less time.

Right.

But if they had just tried to eat 20 per cent less without changing when they ate, they probably would have had trouble sticking to it. I mean, then it would have just been a traditional calorie-cutting diet and those don't usually work, right?

Right. It's just not clear whether the people lost weight because they were eating only during the day or because they were eating less overall.

OK, either way, eating only during the day seems like a good idea, even if all it does is help you eat less overall.

Right.

Fasting

OK, let me ask another question. Even in the mouse study, where the all-day mice and the half-day mice ate the same amount of food overall, it seems like there could be two explanations for why the all-day mice had problems and the half-day mice didn't. Did the all-day mice have problems because they were eating at the wrong times or because they were eating all the time?

I don't understand the question.

Well, it seems like eating all the time can cause problems for two reasons: one is that it will keep my behavior out of sync with my brain clock and the other is that it won't give my cells enough time to do their maintenance. Which of those is actually the problem? I mean, what if I ate only at night? Would I have problems because my behavior and brain clock would be out of sync? Or would I be fine because my cells would still get a long break every day? Obviously, I recognize that this is not practical, I'm just wondering what would happen in theory.

Oh, I see, that's a good question. You're right, from the mouse experiment that I told you about, it's impossible to know whether the half-day mice stayed lean and healthy because their eating was in sync with their brain clock or because they went for long periods each day without eating at all. In fact, there have been *a lot* of other experiments done to try to figure that out:[12] experiments with mice that had a damaged brain clock, mutant mice that had no brain clock at all, mice that were kept in constant light or constant darkness, mice that were forced to eat or be active during one half of the day or the other. Basically, any experiment that you can think of has been done. In the end, it's clear that both eating in sync with your brain clock and taking long breaks from eating are important.

Oh, OK.

But, actually, there's one other set of experiments along these lines that I think we should talk about. There have been a lot experiments that have tried to look only at the effects of taking a long break from

eating by letting animals or people do whatever they want on most days but then giving them almost no food on other days.

Oh, like the 5:2 diet, where you eat whatever you want on five days each week and then fast or eat very little on the other two days?

Yes, exactly.

Does that work?

Well, yes, but it's not exactly clear why. Let me tell you about some experiments.[13]

OK, go ahead.

In the first experiment, researchers raised two groups of mice normally and then kept one group on a normal diet and put the other group on a 10:4 diet.

So the 10:4 mice could eat whatever they wanted for 10 days and then they got very little food for four days?

Right. And the 10:4 mice were kept on that diet for the rest of their lives.

So what happened?

Well, just like in the other experiment with the all-day mice and the half-day mice, the two groups of mice in this experiment ended up eating the same amount of food overall.

So the 10:4 mice ate more on their free days than the normal mice?

Right.

But I suppose the 10:4 mice somehow ended up weighing less than the normal mice?

Oh, yeah. But it wasn't just that. The 10:4 mice were healthier in every way. They even lived 10 per cent longer.

Oh, wow. Why?

Well, it has to be that taking such long breaks from eating gave their cells a lot of time to get their maintenance done.[14]

Right, OK. But I don't think I could go four straight days with very little food. That sounds really hard.

No, me neither. But the 5:2 diet is probably more manageable and the results from experimental studies of humans on the 5:2 diet suggest that it works.[15] Unfortunately, these studies are also hard to interpret because when the people on the 5:2 diet ate very little on two days each week, they didn't make up for it by eating more on their five free days than they would have normally eaten. In fact, they ate less on their free days than they would have normally.

Really? I was always skeptical of the 5:2 diet because I was worried that I would overeat on my free days.

Me too. But, apparently, a lot of people don't. So, it seems like the 5:2 diet works but it's not clear whether it works because it forces people to take a long break from eating to give their cells time to do their maintenance or because they just eat less overall.

Right. But, hold on. Wouldn't a diet like the 5:2 disrupt my daily rhythms? There'd be two days per week when my cells would be expecting me to eat but I wouldn't.

That's true. But your daily rhythms aren't *that* fragile. Actually, the same researchers who did the experiment with the all-day mice and the half-day mice did another experiment where they gave the half-day mice access to food anytime they wanted on the weekends and it didn't seem to disrupt their rhythms too badly.[16]

But did those mice actually eat at random times throughout the day and night on the weekends?

Yes, they did and it didn't seem to do them much harm.

Oh, OK. So it's probably fine to eat at night sometimes.

Of course it is. It's just a bad idea to do it too often.

12
Behavioral change

Personalized advice II

OK, I think I understand why meal timing is important. But it's still not clear to me if I'm better off with a regular routine where I eat at the same times each day to keep my daily rhythms really strong or with a routine like the 5:2 where I eat very little a few days per week to give my cells a long break to do their maintenance.

You're better off with whichever routine you prefer. Arguing about different eating routines is the same as arguing about different mixes of unprocessed foods: maybe some are better than others but it's certainly not clear from the existing evidence. You can find studies that support a lot of different specific routines: a big breakfast and a small dinner,[1] a lot of small meals,[2] fat in the morning and carbs at night[3] – the list goes on and on. The bottom line is that any routine where you eat most of your food during the day and often take long breaks from eating is going to be fine.

OK, I get that, but I still have to choose what and when to eat, so I might as well try to eat the best foods at the best times, right?

What I'm trying to tell you is that, generally speaking, there really are no best foods or best times. As I said, if you look at the average effects of different diets and eating routines across large groups of people, all of them that are a mix of mostly unprocessed foods eaten mostly during the day are equally good. And, again, it may well be that some foods or times are better than others for *you*, but we can never really know that. So all you can do is pick the diet and eating

routine that you think are the best fit for your tastes and schedule and give them a try.

But how do I even know where to start?

Listen, if you're lean and healthy now, you should probably just keep doing what you're doing. But it still might be worth tracking exactly what, when and where you eat for a few weeks.

Why?

Well, if you notice a certain situation in which you eat a lot of processed foods or eat late at night, you could try to find a way to change or avoid it – you never know, it might be easy. When I tracked myself a few years ago, I found that I often ate a pastry at breakfast – you know, like a croissant or a muffin – and that I often had a cookie or a piece of cake with my afternoon coffee.

And you managed to change that?

Yes and no. I was worried that both the breakfast pastries and the afternoon sweets would be very difficult for me to give up, not just because I enjoyed eating them but also because I enjoyed the whole routine that was associated with eating them. I liked going to the café for coffee and a pastry on my way to work in the morning. And I liked taking a break in the afternoon for coffee and sweets.

So what did you do?

Well, it turned out that giving up the breakfast pastries was really easy.

Why?

Because there are so many other eggcellent unprocessed foods to eat for breakfast...

Did you really just say "eggcellent?"

What? No. Anyway, there are so many other excellent unprocessed foods to eat for breakfast. And even though I enjoyed going to the café on my way to work, it was also a little bit stressful because I always had to squeeze onto a packed subway train afterwards. Now I eat at home and get on the train earlier, which is much more comfortable. So my new breakfast routine is both more enjoyable and healthier.

Great. And what about the afternoon sweets?

I still haven't given those up.

Why not?

I don't know, it's just too hard for me. I mean, what else am I going to have with my coffee?

I don't know. Fruit?

Are you serious? Fruit and coffee? I don't think so.

But don't you have fruit and coffee together at breakfast?

That's different.

Why?

Because it's breakfast!

Oh, right, I see.

Anyway, I'm sticking with my afternoon sweets because I can. The rest of my diet is good enough that I can get away with it. I'm not trying to win a prize for being the world's healthiest eater. In fact, all I'm trying to do is live a long and happy life. I know that I have to stay lean and healthy in order to do that but I'm not going to give up things I enjoy if I don't have to.

OK, fair enough.

And I do think that having my afternoon sweets helps me avoid eating other processed foods. My pleasure system knows it's going to get its way each afternoon and that seems to be enough to get it to behave itself the rest of the time. On most days, my afternoon sweets are really the only processed food I eat.

Really?

Sure. I mean, breakfast is easy, right? Eggs, either alone or with some vegetables mixed in, whole grain cereal with milk, yogurt, fruit, nuts, avocados, raw fish . . .

Yeah, breakfast is easy.

Dinner is also pretty easy if you cook. I usually just have a piece of meat or fish with a pile of vegetables on the side and some fruit for dessert. I guess lunch can be trickier but it's easy for me because I have a lot of great lunch options where I live and work.

OK, so you think having the afternoon sweets every day is what allows you to stick to unprocessed foods the rest of the time?

I think that the afternoon sweets work really well for me but they might be disastrous for someone else. I have trouble going a whole day without sweets but I have no problem eating just one cookie or a small piece of cake and then stopping. I'm sure there are other people who can easily go a whole day without sweets but are more likely to end up overdoing it whenever they do eat them. For someone like that, it might better to avoid sweets entirely during the week and eat them only on the weekends or something like that.

Right. So what you're saying is that you can't really help me improve my eating without knowing a lot more about me.

Well, I can tell you to eat mostly unprocessed foods and to eat mostly during the day. But, as we've established, that's a lot easier said than done and the strategies that work for other people may not work for you at all. If you track yourself over a few weeks, I'm sure you'll be able to come up with some that might.

You make it sound so easy.

Well, honestly, I do find it to be easy. I mean, I have some clear advantages: I live in a place where unprocessed foods are easy to find and I have enough money to afford them. Maybe I'm also just lucky. Maybe my genes make it easier for me to deal with all the things about the modern environment that are causing problems for other people.[4] But I'm not sure about that. I actually have a lot of trouble resisting tasty foods when they're right in front of me. I think the reason I'm able to stick to a diet of mostly unprocessed foods is that I've developed a deliberate approach to eating that takes advantage of my strengths and protects me from my weaknesses.

What do you mean?

Well, for example, I know that I have a weakness for sweets. Basically, if I see them, I'm going to eat them. On the other hand, I'm a good shopper: if I go with a list, I'll stick to it. So I have a rule that I can only buy the sweets I'm going to eat that afternoon. That way, there are never any sweets around the house after dinner.

But you could just go out and get more sweets after dinner, right?

Right, but I don't.

Why not?

Because it's inconvenient. Apparently, the time and effort that it would take for me to go out and buy something after dinner are enough to stop me from going.

I see.

But this approach only works for me because I'm a good shopper. It wouldn't work at all for someone who loses control when they shop and ends up with a lot of things they don't need. Someone like that might want to try to get their groceries delivered or get someone else to do their shopping for them.

OK, hold on, now you're starting to sound like some article on the internet. You know, "10 ways to effortlessly melt away the pounds."

What do you mean?

Well, I always see tips like "Don't keep sweets in the house" or "Don't shop when you're hungry," but none of those things really help, do they?

Oh, they certainly can. Why are you so skeptical?

I don't know, I guess they sound too simple.

Well, I don't think something needs to be complicated in order to work. Tips like that are based on the idea that unhealthy eating is ultimately about being unable to resist processed foods, which, when it comes down to it, is just true.

So we're back to being animals with no control over ourselves?

Why do you have such a big problem with that? Just because we put a man on the moon, everything about us has to be complicated? I'm sorry, but that doesn't make any sense. The reason that so many people are overweight is not complicated: we've created an environment with processed foods that are unnaturally tasty, unnaturally free of fiber and unnaturally abundant, but we're stuck with bodies and brains that are designed for an environment with unprocessed foods that are bland, full of fiber and scarce. Sure, there are plenty of other factors that can makes things worse – stress, lack of sleep, cultural pressures and so on – but if there weren't processed foods everywhere, it's pretty unlikely that those other factors alone would be making people gain weight.

OK, OK, calm down.

Sorry. What is definitely complicated, however, is figuring out how to stay lean and healthy in our modern environment. And a lot of what makes that so complicated is the fact that we're all different from each other: we all have different genes, different tastes, different lifestyles, different cultures and different resources, so there's never going to be a one-size-fits-all solution. We're all trying to achieve the same thing – finding a healthy diet and eating routine we can actually stick to – but the best way to achieve it is going to be different for each of us.

Simple strategies

And you think simple strategies can help?

Sure. Anything that makes it easier for you to resist eating processed foods can help. One way to avoid making bad decisions is to avoid making any decisions at all. So something as simple as keeping all of your foods in closed cabinets can be extremely powerful: if you don't notice them, you won't have to decide not to eat them.

Out of sight, out of mind, right?

Exactly. I know it sounds simple but that kind of idea can go a long way. There have been a lot of studies showing how powerful the "out of sight, out of mind" concept can be.[5] For example, researchers took a group of people and gave each one a bowl of candy to put on their desk every day for four weeks.[6] On half of the days, the bowl was clear but on the other half of the days, the bowl was opaque.

So on half of the days, the people could see the candy and on the other half of the days they couldn't?

Right. And, on average, they ate almost twice as much candy on the days when they could see it.

Wow.

Yeah. And the same kind of effect has been found in a lot of different studies. If you track yourself for a few weeks, I guarantee you'll notice that you have unplanned snacks just because you happened to see a particular food or something that reminds you of it. And if you find that your unplanned snacking often happens in a particular situation, you should be able to find a way to prevent it.

If it's something as simple as walking into the kitchen and seeing the cookie jar, you can just get rid of the cookie jar or put it inside a cabinet or replace it with a fruit bowl.

That sounds easy enough.

Well, the cookie jar example is a simple one. It's possible that the important factors in the situations that trigger your unplanned snacking might be harder to identify – maybe you always end up snacking after you have a meeting with your boss or something like that – but, if you can identify the important factors, you should be able to think of a way to change them.

But what if the factors aren't entirely under my control? I mean, the rest of my family may not want to see the cookie jar go.

Well, I hope that you'd be able to sell them the benefits of getting rid of the cookie jar, both for them and for you. But, whatever situations you identify, you probably won't even need to change them completely. It may be enough just to make snacking a bit more inconvenient. For example, in the same study that I just told you about with the candy bowls, just moving the clear bowl to another table a few metres away – but still in sight – had almost the same effect as making the bowl opaque. So whatever changes you're trying to make, you can probably find a way to make them without bothering other people too much.

I see. OK, I think I will track myself like you're suggesting. If nothing else, I think it would be interesting to see what kinds of situations lead me to eat unplanned snacks.

Good. You should also try to identify any situations that lead you to overeat – I mean, situations that lead you to eat more than you intended to when you started the meal. Again, I think you'll find that you often overeat in particular situations. Maybe it's when you watch TV or when you've had alcohol before dinner or when you serve the meal "family style."

What do you mean "family style?"

I mean when you just put all of the food on the dinner table and then let everyone serve themselves. That can be a dangerous situation because it makes it very easy to keep refilling your plate.

Right. But I guess that's an easy situation to avoid. I can just serve the food in the kitchen and only take the plates to the dinner table, right?

Sure. Simply having to get up and go to the kitchen might be enough to prevent you from overeating. And, if it's not, there are plenty of other things you can try: you can make sure to only cook enough for one serving or you can package leftovers and put them in the fridge before you even start eating.[7] I'm sure you'll be able to figure something out. The key is to make good decisions before a meal in order to avoid making bad decisions during it.

OK, hold on, let's take a step back. You started off by spending a lot of time telling me about all the systems in my body and brain that try to help me match the number of calories that I eat and burn – you know, assuming that my leptin is working properly, my brain will adjust how hungry I am, how active I am, how much I fidget and how much energy my cells waste by creating heat to keep me at my natural weight, right?

Right...

And if I remember correctly, you even got angry with me for questioning how effective those systems were.

Oh, c'mon, I didn't get angry with you.

Either way, now it seems like you're telling me that these systems aren't really that important. I mean, if something as simple as hiding the cookie jar is really going to have an effect on my weight, my weight regulation systems can't really be all that effective, right?

OK, I see your point. If you're lean and healthy, and your weight regulation systems are working properly, it's likely that these strategies for avoiding unplanned snacking and overeating may not have any effect. Even if you do manage to lose weight by hiding the cookie jar, your brain will notice that you're underweight and it will make you hungry or tired or tell your cells to waste less energy and you'll end up back at your natural weight one way or another. On the other hand, the systems that try to match the calories that you eat and burn obviously aren't perfect. For example, we talked about how the calories in sugar and drinks don't get counted properly. So all the things we've been discussing – eating mostly unprocessed foods, eating mostly during the day and avoiding situations in which you're likely to eat unplanned snacks or overeat – are all ways that you can make it easier for your metabolic and weight regulation systems to do their jobs.

Losing weight

OK, so the strategies that we've been discussing for avoiding unplanned snacks and overeating might only help a little bit if I'm lean and healthy but what if I'm already overweight? Would they be a lot more helpful then?

Definitely. I mean, if you're overweight and your immune cells are interfering with your insulin and your leptin, your weight regulation systems definitely aren't working properly and you need all the help that you can get, right?

OK, so what would you do if you were overweight?

Well, I can tell you what I wouldn't do: I wouldn't try any kind of traditional diet where I eat very little and attempt to lose weight quickly.

Why not?

Because that kind of diet hardly ever works.

What do you mean?

I mean that even if you lose weight initially, you're probably just going to gain it back and end up overweight again.[8] It's always the same: you lose weight quickly and easily in the beginning but then your weight loss slows down and it becomes harder and harder to stick to the diet and eventually you just go back to your old ways and your old weight. All that stress and sacrifice only to end up back where you started. It's sad.

Yeah, you're right. I know a lot of people who keep going through that cycle. Why is it that weight loss always slows down as a diet goes on?

For a few reasons. First of all, a lot of the weight that you lose when you start a diet is just water. Do you remember why you store most of your energy as fat rather than as glucose?

Because fat packs together well but glucose doesn't, right?

Right. If you want to pack glucose together for storage, you have to add water. Now, while most of your stored energy is fat, you do also store some glucose.

Right. My liver will store some of the glucose that I eat during the day and release it to keep my brain going at night, right?

Right. And your muscles will actually store some as well. But when you start a diet and go a few days without eating much, all of that glucose will get released from storage. And when you release your glucose from storage, the water that was stored with it gets released as well.

Oh, OK, I didn't know that. I've heard people talk about "water weight" but I didn't really know what it was. So that's why it's so easy to lose a lot of weight quickly at the beginning of a diet?

Right. And, of course, as soon as you start eating normally and storing glucose again, that water weight will immediately come back.

Right.

But there are also several other reasons why weight loss slows down as a diet goes on. One is very simple: as you lose more and more weight, you need fewer and fewer calories just to maintain your weight.[9]

Right. So if I want to keep losing weight, I need to keep eating less and less, right?

Right. Let's say you're overweight and you need 2,500 calories per day just to maintain your weight. If you start eating 2,400 calories per day, you're not just going to keep losing weight forever until you disappear, right?

No, I'm going to lose a few pounds and then stay at whatever weight requires 2,400 calories per day to maintain.

Exactly. So if you want to keep losing weight, then you need to drop down to 2,300 calories per day and then 2,200, and so on, which is not going to be easy.

Right.

But the biggest reason why weight loss slows down as a diet goes on is that your weight regulation systems are going to work against you.[10] If your immune cells are interfering with your insulin and leptin then your brain is going to think that you are below your natural weight already and it's going to do everything it can to stop you from losing even more.

Right. I'll normally burn hundreds of extra calories automatically by fidgeting or wasting energy as heat. But if my brain thinks that I'm below my natural weight and I save those calories instead, I'll have to either exercise more or eat less to make up for it. And doing either of those things is going to be very difficult, because, again, my immune cells are interfering with my leptin, which means that my self-control system will be much weaker than it should be.

Right. It's hard enough to stay lean when our weight regulation systems are working properly. Once they start working against us, well...

OK, well, I guess it's easy to see why most diets fail.

Yeah, it's not exactly surprising. And yet we still beat ourselves up about it. Being overweight is not something to be ashamed of. It doesn't make you a bad person. In fact, for millions of years, having a strong drive to seek and eat food was a big advantage because food was scarce. Now, all of the sudden, food is everywhere and we blame ourselves for eating it? It's really perverse.

So you're saying that if I'm overweight, it's not really my fault?

Well, it may not be your fault but it is still your problem. The fact is that having a strong drive to seek and eat food has become a disadvantage. Recognizing that you are overweight because of a mismatch between your genes and your environment, rather than some character flaw, is helpful but it doesn't solve the problem. It's still up to you to figure out how to overcome that disadvantage.

But if our environment is such a big problem, why don't we just change it?

That's exactly what all of these little strategies for avoiding unplanned snacking and overeating are designed to do. Obviously you can't control everything about your environment but you can control the places where you spend most of your time – you know, like your home and your office. If you want to give yourself the best chance to lose weight, you need to try to transform your local environment from one with convenient, processed foods to one with inconvenient, unprocessed foods. If your big problem is unplanned snacking, changing your environment might help a lot.

And what if my problem is overeating at planned meals?

Then I guess you'd need to get really aggressive about portion control. There are plenty of strategies you can try, like getting smaller plates and bowls or repacking all of your food into single servings or decreasing the variety of your individual meals. There have been

a lot studies showing that strategies like that can make people eat a lot less without even noticing.[11] Of course, there's no guarantee that something like that will work but there's no harm in trying. Or you could even try one of those programs that provides all of the meals for you.

Does that work?

It can.[12] Programs like that are good because they take a lot of the decision making out of eating. And they also provide a community for support, which can help a lot. But, honestly, if I were trying to lose weight, I would just start off slow and try things that I thought would be easy at first.

Is that really going to get me anywhere?

It might, you never know. And given that a traditional diet is unlikely to get you anywhere, I don't see the harm in trying something else first. We have this idea that weight-loss strategies have to be difficult to be effective. And, of course, that's true in general. If you do something really easy, like continue to overeat and remain inactive, you won't lose any weight. If you do something really difficult, like starve yourself and run marathons, you will. But it's also true that different things will be hard or easy for different people. It was easy for me to give up breakfast pastries and hard for me to give up afternoon sweets but for someone else it might be the exact opposite. So I would start with what I thought would be easy for me and work from there. At least then I'd be developing an approach that I could actually stick to. I mean, what good is losing weight if you're just going to put it back on again? That kind of cycle is actually really stressful and frustrating.[13]

I see what you mean. It's the same with different foods, right? In general, it might be true that processed foods taste better than unprocessed foods but different people have different tastes.

Exactly. In some cases, you might even be able to replace processed foods with unprocessed foods that you actually prefer. Like I said, part of the reason it was easy for me to give up breakfast pastries was that I really enjoy a lot of other unprocessed breakfast foods. If I was trying to lose weight, I would make sure that everything I ate – processed or unprocessed – was something that I really enjoyed. That way, I'd always be keeping my pleasure system as happy as possible and saving my self-control system for the times when I really needed it. It's important to have some variety, of course, but there are so many different foods. You should be able to find plenty that you like, so there is really no point in eating any that you don't.

Yeah, that makes sense.

Exercise II

And, of course, if I was trying to lose weight, I would exercise *a lot*.

Right. Because exercise doesn't just burn calories, it also reduces inflammation directly, right?

That's right. But there's a lot more to it than that.

Like what?

Actually, we still don't know all of the reasons why exercise is so beneficial. The benefits of exercise – in terms of reducing the risk of a heart attack or a stroke or something like that – are about double what you would predict based on how much weight loss the exercise causes or how much it decreases inflammation.[14] So there is clearly a lot more going on.

I see. But the biggest benefit of exercise is still just the fact that it burns a lot of calories, right?

Right, and, in particular, it burns fat. If you want to lose weight, you have to burn the fat that is stored in your fat cells rather than just the glucose and fat that are already in your blood. One way to do that is to go for long periods without eating.

Right, because my blood glucose will be low, which means my insulin will be low, so my fat cells will start releasing fat rather than storing it.

Exactly. That's one of the reasons why it's good to eat mostly during the day. If you eat dinner early, then a lot of the energy your body uses when you're sleeping will have to come from your fat cells, rather than from food.

Right.

The other way to burn the fat that is stored in your fat cells is to exercise. When you exercise, your muscles need a lot of energy.[15] They'll start by using whatever glucose and fat are already in your blood,

as well as the little bit of glucose that they have stored. But that's probably not going to be enough. Your brain knows your muscles are going to need a lot of energy so it releases the stress hormone adrenaline, which tells your fat cells to start releasing fat and tells your liver to start making and releasing glucose.

Right, I remember.

And the longer you exercise, the more fat you will burn. Once your muscles use up the glucose and fat already in your blood, and the glucose they have stored, they'll have to depend entirely on glucose from your liver and fat from your fat cells. The amount of glucose your liver can make and release is limited so, as you exercise for longer and longer, your muscles will have no choice but to burn more and more fat from your fat cells.

I see.

And, actually, even after you're done exercising, you'll still burn more calories, and more fat, over the next day or two than you normally would.[16]

Why?

Well, you'll burn more fat than normal simply because some of the glucose you eat will be put back into storage in your muscles and liver. And you'll burn more calories than normal because your cells will be doing a lot of repair and improvement work.

Like making my muscles bigger?

Right. I mean, it's not so much about making things bigger, it's more about making them better. Your body responds to exercise by making changes to help glucose and fat get to your cells more quickly and also to help your cells process them more quickly once they get there.[17]

Oh, right, I remember now. One way to get fat to my cells more quickly is to build more blood vessels in between my fat cells so they can release fat more easily. And that's helpful not only for exercise but also for reducing inflammation.

That's right. Do you remember why?

Because part of the problem with overeating and gaining weight is that my fat cells keep growing and some of them end up far away from any blood vessels. If things get really bad, some of my fat cells will start dying because they don't get enough oxygen and my immune cells will notice and take action. But if I build more blood vessels in between my fat cells, that's less likely to happen.

Exactly. And the changes that help your cells process glucose and fat more quickly are also really important.

Why? Oh, because those changes are also helpful for reducing inflammation, right? If they leave my cells better prepared to process glucose and fat in general, that means there will be less of a build-up of waste and half-processed glucose and fat when I overeat, so I'll have less backlog-driven inflammation.

Very good. And, as we discussed, exercise also decreases inflammation directly.

Right, because exercise also causes my brain to release the other stress hormone cortisol, which decreases inflammation.

Right, that's a big part of it. But your muscles also release their own hormones to decrease inflammation.

Oh, muscles release hormones too?

Sure. And they can have really strong effects.[18] Let me tell you about an experiment.[19]

Go ahead.

OK, so researchers took rats and overfed them for a few months until they became overweight, inflamed, and insulin and leptin resistant. Then they split the rats into two groups: one group that just stayed in their normal cages and another group that was forced to exercise.

How did they force the second group to exercise?

They put them into water so they no choice but to swim for a while.

Oh, OK.

So then, after one group exercised and the other group didn't, the researchers kept track of how much food the rats ate over the next 12 hours.

And?

The rats that exercised actually ate a lot less than the rats that didn't.

What? Why? Shouldn't they have eaten more to make up for the calories they burned during the exercise?

Well, the researchers did a lot of other experiments to figure out what was going on. In the end, they found that the reason that the rats ate less after exercise was because the hormones released by their muscles decreased their inflammation.

But why did decreasing their inflammation make them eat less?

Because it temporarily stopped the immune cells in their brains from interfering with their insulin and leptin.

Oh, the hormones from their muscles made it all the way into their brains?

Yes, and they had strong effects on the immune cells there. So the exercise actually made the rats' weight-regulation systems work properly again, at least for a while. Instead of thinking that the rats were below their natural weight because their leptin wasn't working, their brains were able to see that they were actually overweight and made them less hungry.

Oh, I get it. If I'm overweight and inflammation is disrupting my metabolic and weight-regulation systems, I can use exercise to make those systems temporarily work properly again. So exercising a lot won't just help me burn more calories, it will also help me eat less.

That's the idea. And there do seem to be some studies of obese humans which support the idea that exercise does decrease appetite.[20] And, of course, the hormones released by your muscles don't just go to your brain, they go everywhere and decrease inflammation all over your body. For example, exercise even decreases the amount of inflammation caused by bits of dead bacteria that get into your blood from your intestines.[21]

Really. Wow. OK, so if I want to lose weight I should definitely exercise as much as possible.

Right.

OK, so what's the best exercise plan? Should I just try to do a little bit of cardio every day? Or should I try to lift weights a few times per week?

You know what I'm going to say by now.

Oh, right. The best exercise plan is the one that I enjoy the most because that's the one that I'll actually stick to.

Yup. Now, I'm not trying to say that all exercises are equally effective. Prolonged, low-intensity exercises like jogging will probably help you burn more fat and lose more weight than short, high-intensity exercises like weight lifting.[22]

Why?

Because, as I said before, you really start burning a lot of fat after you use up the glucose that was already in your blood or stored in your muscles. If you only do short bouts of exercise, you may never get to that point.

Oh, right.

But, on the other hand, inflammation seems to decrease much more after high-intensity exercise than it does after low-intensity exercise.[23]

Oh. So then I guess the best plan would probably combine prolonged, low-intensity exercise to burn fat with short, high-intensity exercise to decrease inflammation.

Probably. But comparing different exercise plans is just like comparing different mixes of foods or eating routines: some may be better for you than others but there is no way of really knowing until you try them.

Right.

And, anyway, even more than with choosing foods or eating routines, choosing exercises that you actually enjoy is critical. There is no point in forcing yourself to jog if you really hate it, because you're not going to stick with it. And you're not just going to start jogging more slowly or for less time, you're going to quit altogether.

But what if my weight regulation systems are making it miserable for me to exercise because my immune cells are interfering with my leptin and my brain thinks that I'm below my natural weight? Am I really going to be able to find any exercise I enjoy?

Maybe. The only way to find out is to try. I've tried *a lot* of different kinds of exercise in my life and I've been amazed at how much I enjoy some and hate others. For example, I think I could play squash or basketball all day long and love every minute of it. But jogging is almost impossible for me: whenever I try to jog, all I can think about is how much I hate it and I end up stopping pretty quickly. If I'd only ever tried jogging – or biking or swimming or any other kind of pure cardio – I would probably think that I hated all exercise. But, fortunately, I tried a lot of other things and found plenty of them that I like.

Right.

But if I was overweight and just trying to get started with exercise, I would definitely ease into it. I would just start by walking every day. And I'd be very careful not to overdo it at first. What you really want is for exercise to become a regular part of your daily routine – you know, something that you just kind of do each day, rather than something that you have to make a decision to do each day.[24]

Sure, that would be great, but it's wishful thinking, isn't it?

Not if you enjoy the exercise. And if the exercise itself isn't enjoyable enough, you need to try other ways to make it enjoyable. For example, you could try walking with other people that you like to talk to. Or listening to podcasts or audio books.

Or walking on a treadmill with a TV.

Exactly. If you're the kind of person who gets sucked into binge-watching TV shows, you could take advantage of that to keep yourself exercising. You know how it works: if your pleasure system learns that getting on the treadmill and turning on the TV leads to the release of opioids and cannabinoids, then it will release dopamine to make sure that you do it. Whether the pleasure comes from the exercise itself or something else related to it doesn't really matter.

Right. So you've managed to make exercise a part of your daily routine?

Sort of. My routine is more weekly than daily. For example, I play squash with the same group of friends every Monday night. And it's not a decision I make each week. I don't have to check my schedule or clear it with my family. It's just a given. The same way I leave home to go to work every Monday morning, I leave work to go to squash every Monday night. And because I'm not really making a decision about whether or not to go, I never stop to think about how tired I am or anything like that. But even if I was tired and didn't really feel like playing squash, I'd probably go and play because I look forward to seeing my friends.

Counting calories

Right, OK. So let's say that I find some good eating and exercise routines that I can actually stick to. If I want to lose weight, how many extra calories should I try to burn per day?

What do you mean?

Well, if I want to lose weight, I have to burn more calories than I eat, right? You said a pound of fat was 3,000 calories?

3,500.

Right, 3,500. So if I want to lose a pound per week, then I have to burn... let's see... 500 more calories per day than I eat. So shouldn't I track the number of calories that I eat and burn to make sure that I'm maintaining that 500-calorie difference?

How are you going to do that?

How am I going to do what?

Track the number of calories that you eat and burn.

I don't know. Is it really that hard? There are calorie counts on food labels, right?

OK, first of all, the numbers on labels are way off.[25] In fact, they're allowed to be: the law allows a margin of error up to 20 per cent. So something that says 500 calories on it might actually be 400 or 600. But that doesn't even matter.

Why not?

Because most unprocessed foods aren't going to have labels on them.

Oh, right. But I could weigh everything, right?

You could, but that isn't going to get you an accurate calorie count either. And even if you could find a way to measure how many calories you eat, you have absolutely no chance of accurately measuring how many calories you burn.

Why not?

How are you going to do it?

Well, if I know my height, weight, age, percent body fat and all that, can't I calculate how many calories I'll burn during a particular exercise? Isn't that what fancy treadmills do?

C'mon.

What?

You know that you can burn a different number of calories from the same amount of activity depending on whether your cells are

saving or wasting energy. How is your treadmill going to account for that?

I don't know.

And even if you could measure the calories you burned while exercising, you'd still only solve a small part of the problem. You burn most of your calories when you're just sitting around.[26]

You mean because of fidgeting and stuff like that?

Yes. But also just staying warm and keeping your organs going. The only way to really measure how many calories you eat and burn in a day is to lock yourself up in an air-tight lab with some very expensive equipment. And even then, the accuracy of the measurements would only be barely enough to be useful.[27]

So counting calories is pointless.

Counting calories inaccurately is pointless because it's only going to mislead you. But that doesn't mean you shouldn't keep track of anything. First of all, you have to keep track of your weight. If you keep losing weight slowly and steadily over time, you know that you can just keep doing whatever you're doing. On the other hand, if you go a month or two without losing weight, you know that you have to try something else. And if you want to be at least a little bit systematic about trying different strategies, then you also have keep track of your eating and exercising.

But not in terms of calories?

No.

So something like "today I walked two miles in 30 minutes," rather than "today, I burned 300 calories while walking."

Exactly.

What about for eating?

You could keep track of how many unplanned snacks you have each day and how many times you eat more than you intend to and how many of your meals and snacks contain processed foods.

I see. And if I'm not losing weight then I know that I need to either increase the exercise or decrease the unplanned snacks, overeating and processed foods.

Right. Keeping track of your eating and exercising that way is going to be much more effective than trying to count calories.

OK, so is it fair to say that we know enough to be confident about some general guidelines – eat a mix of mostly unprocessed foods, eat mostly during the day and exercise a lot – but we're not really sure about much beyond that?

Yes, I think that's fair. You're never going to be able to figure out exactly which mix of foods or exercises is best for you. Maybe someday you'll be able to get some tests to find out, but not yet. And, anyway, any differences in the health benefits of different foods or exercises are probably going to be small compared to the differences in how much you enjoy them.

Right. And if I don't enjoy a particular food or exercise, it doesn't really matter how healthy it is because I won't stick with it.

Right. So just make sure that you follow the general guidelines and try not to worry too much about the details. If you want to worry about the details of something, it should be your environment. If you can figure out exactly what triggers your unplanned snacking or your overeating, and find a way to change it, that's going to be much more helpful than trying any particular mix of foods or exercises.

The end

Right. So is that it, then?

Pretty much.

Good, I'm starving. Do you want to get dinner?

Sure, where?

I don't know, McDonald's?

What?

Just kidding!

Notes

Chapter 1

1 In fact, there are backup plans for the backup plans. For a detailed overview of how the body attempts to survive starvation, see McCue (2010).
2 For a detailed overview of how insulin controls the movement of fat in and out of fat cells, see Duncan et al. (2007).
3 Berger et al., 2015.

Chapter 2

1 For a detailed overview of how fructose can cause liver damage, see Lustig (2013).
2 Bellentani et al., 2010; Lazo et al., 2013.
3 Ng et al., 2014.
4 For a detailed discussion of the evolutionary mismatch idea, see Power and Schulkin (2013).
5 Björck et al., 1994.
6 Ludwig et al., 1999; Pawlak et al., 2004; Walsh et al., 2013.
7 For a detailed discussion of the idea that weight gain is caused by recurring insulin overshoots, see Taubes (2010).
8 For a detailed overview of the consequences of inflamed fat, see Gregor and Hotamisligil (2011).
9 For a detailed overview of what happens when cells get overwhelmed by glucose or fat, see Hotamisligil (2010).
10 For a detailed overview of the causes and consequences of insulin resistance, see Olefsky and Glass (2010) or Odegaard and Chawla (2013).
11 Lumeng et al., 2007.
12 For a detailed overview of how inflammation causes diabetes, see Donath and Shoelson (2011).
13 For a detailed overview of how inflammation causes the formation of plaques, see Rocha and Libby (2009).
14 Musunuru, 2010.
15 For a description of the composition of liver fat packages before and after depletion, see Sniderman et al. (2001).
16 For a detailed overview of how inflammation changes liver fat packages, see Choi and Ginsberg (2011).
17 Adiels et al., 2008.
18 Packard, 2003.
19 For a detailed overview of how small depleted liver fat packages are created, see Sniderman et al. (2001) or Tchernof and Després (2013).

Chapter 3

1 For a detailed overview of the nerves that connect the gut and the brain, see Brookes et al. (2013).
2 For a detailed overview of the different gut hormones, see Wren and Bloom (2007).

3 For a detailed overview of ghrelin, see Gil-Campos et al. (2006) or Massadi et al. (2014).

4 For a detailed overview of the different hormones released by fat cells, see Ouchi et al. (2011).

5 Kohno et al., 2003.

6 For a detailed overview of the pleasure system, see Berridge and Kringelbach (2015) or Kenny (2011).

7 For a detailed overview of opioids and cannabinoids, see Cota et al. (2006), Le Merrer et al. (2009) or Parsons and Hurd (2015).

8 For a detailed overview of dopamine, see Berridge and Kringelbach (2015), Glimcher (2011) or Wise (2004).

9 O'Connor et al., 2015.

10 Hommel et al., 2006.

11 For a detailed overview of how the self-control system inhibits behaviors, see Aron (2007).

12 For a detailed overview of the balance between the pleasure and self-control systems, see Inzlicht et al. (2014).

13 Baicy et al., 2007.

14 For a discussion of the similarities between food and drug addiction, see DiLeone et al. (2012) or Garber and Lustig (2011).

15 Guo et al., 2014; Karlsson et al., 2015.

16 DelParigi et al., 2006.

17 Dallman et al., 2003.

18 For a detailed overview of the stress system, see Adam and Epel (2007) or McEwen et al. (2015).

19 Schwabe et al., 2010.

20 Butts et al., 2011; Piazza et al., 1996.

21 For a detailed overview of the long-term effects of stress on the brain, see Arnsten (2015).

22 Dallman et al., 2003.

23 For a detailed overview of the differences between belly fat and other fat, see Ibrahim (2010).

24 Nielsen et al., 2004.

25 For a detailed overview of the consequences of brain inflammation, see Ryan et al. (2012).

26 For a detailed overview of leptin resistance, see Myers et al. (2012). The basics are clear but a lot of the details are still being worked out – see Myers (2015).

27 Zhang et al., 2008.

Chapter 4

1 One gram of fat contains about nine calories (Livesey and Elia, 1988).

2 For a detailed overview of the relationship between genetics and body weight, see Barsh et al. (2000).

3 Levine et al., 1999; Levine et al., 2005.

4 Levine et al., 2005.

5 For a detailed overview of how the brain controls fidgeting, see Kotz et al. (2008).

6 For a detailed overview of how cells can use more or less energy, see Liesa and Shirihai (2013).

7 Major et al., 2007

8 For a detailed overview of how the hypothalamus controls the amount of energy that cells waste, see Yang and Ruan (2015).

9 Dombrowski et al., 2014; Fildes et al., 2015; Kraschnewski et al., 2010; Mann et al., 2007.

10 For a detailed overview of why it is so hard to lose weight and keep it off, see MacLean et al. (2011), Ochner et al. (2013), or Rosenbaum and Leibel (2010).

11 Fernandes et al., 2015; Morton et al., 2011.

12 For a detailed overview of how exercise can be pleasurable, see Garland et al. (2011).

13 Boecker et al., 2008.

14 Robinson and Berridge, 2013.

15 For a detailed overview of how exercise can decrease inflammation, see Gleeson et al. (2011) or Lancaster and Febbraio (2014).

16 Miller et al., 2008.

17 For a detailed overview of the benefits of exercise, see Hawley et al. (2014).

Chapter 5

1 For a detailed overview of gut bacteria, see Clemente et al. (2012), Hooper et al. (2012), Nicholson et al. (2012) or Tremaroli and Bäckhed (2012).
2 Whitman et al., 1998.
3 This number is just an estimate; see Sender et al. (2016).
4 For a detailed overview of fiber fat, see den Besten et al. (2013) or Sonnenburg and Sonnenburg (2014).
5 For a detailed overview of the leaky gut problem, see Bischoff et al. (2014).
6 Morton et al., 2014.
7 For an overview of studies that have measured the benefits of fiber consumption, see Aune et al. (2016).
8 Powley and Phillips, 2004.
9 For a detailed overview of the effects of fiber on hunger, see Slavin (2013).
10 Goodrich et al., 2014.
11 Stephen and Cummings, 1980.
12 Turnbaugh et al., 2006.
13 David et al., 2013.
14 For a detailed overview of the vitamins made by gut bacteria, see LeBlanc et al. (2013).
15 For a detailed overview of how gut bacteria communicate with the brain, see Collins et al. (2012) or Cryan and Dinan (2012).
16 Nwokolo et al. (2003).
17 For a detailed overview of how gut bacteria change over time, see Lozupone et al. (2012).
18 For a detailed overview of the consequences of antibiotic-driven changes in gut bacteria, see Blaser (2014) or Cox and Blaser (2015).
19 Dethlefsen and Relman, 2011.
20 Ley et al., 2008.

Chapter 6

1 For a detailed overview of how smoking causes cancer, see Hecht (1999).
2 Just to be clear, you should worry about smoking (Jha, 2009).
3 For a list of approved additives, see http://www.fda.gov/Food/IngredientsPackaging Labeling/FoodAdditivesIngredients (USA) or https://www.food.gov.uk/science/ additives (EU).
4 Chassaing et al. (2015).
5 Suez et al. (2014).
6 For a detailed overview of the food additive approval process in the USA, see Neltner et al. (2013).
7 For a detailed overview of the effects of pesticides on human health, see Alavanja et al. (2004), Gilden et al. (2010) or Sanborn et al. (2007).
8 For a detailed overview of worldwide pesticide usage, see http://www.epa.gov/pesticides/ pesticides-industry-sales-and-usage-2006-and-2007-market-estimates.
9 For a summary of the studies examining pesticide contamination in food, see Smith-Spangler et al. (2012).
10 Colborn, 2006.
11 Bouchard et al., 2010.
12 Schoenfeld and Ioannidis, 2013.
13 Klümper and Qaim, 2014.
14 For a summary of the studies examining the health effects of GM foods, see DeFrancesco, (2013).
15 Oldroyd, 2007.
16 For a list of approved organic additives, see http://www.ams.usda.gov/rules-regulations/ organic/ national-list (USA) or http://www.faia.org.uk/food-choices/organic-food (EU).
17 Dangour et al., 2010.

Chapter 7

1   Cromwell, 2002.
2   Cho et al., 2012; Cox et al., 2014.
3   For a detailed overview of how gut bacteria interact with the immune system, see Garrett et al. (2010), Hooper et al. (2012) or Lee and Mazmanian (2010).
4   Bersaglieri et al., 2004.
5   Mazmanian et al., 2005.
6   For a detailed overview of the relationship between gut bacteria and IBD, see Manichanh et al. (2012).
7   Arpaia et al., 2013; Maslowski et al., 2009; Smith et al., 2013.
8   Bashir et al., 2004; Hill et al., 2012; Stefka et al., 2014; Trompette et al., 2014.
9   Kaprio et al., 1992.
10 Burrows et al., 2015; Wen et al., 2008.
11 Knip and Siljander (2016).
12 For a detailed overview of how gut bacteria interact with immune cells, see Garrett et al. (2010) or Thaiss et al. (2016).
13 Elinav et al., 2011; Henao-Mejia et al., 2012; Vijay-Kumar et al., 2010.
14 Abrams et al., 1963.
15 For a detailed overview of how gut bacteria interact with intestinal wall cells, see Ulluwishewa et al. (2011).
16 Dethlefsen and Relman, 2011.
17 Mikkelsen et al., 2015.
18 Laxminarayan et al., 2013.
19 http://usda.mannlib.cornell.edu/MannUsda/viewDocumentInfo.do?documentID=1497.
20 Seufert et al., 2012.

Chapter 8

1   For a detailed overview of the health risks associated with trans fats, see Mozaffarian et al. (2006).
2   Siri-Tarino et al., 2010.
3   For a discussion of the history of trans fats, see Schleifer (2012).
4   Mauger et al., 2003.
5   Lopez-Garcia et al., 2005; Mozaffarian et al., 2004.
6   Lee et al., 2001; Shi et al., 2006.
7   Shi et al., 2006.
8   Milanski et al., 2009.
9   Ghoshal et al., 2008; Laugerette et al., 2011.
10 Cani et al., 2007, 2008; Everard et al., 2013.
11 Caesar et al., 2015.
12 For a detailed overview of how difficult it is to know what people actually eat, see Winkler (2005).
13 Emmons et al., 1994; Palaniappan et al., 2001; Troisi et al., 1991.
14 Chowdhury et al., 2014; de Souza et al., 2015.
15 Bryan et al., 2012.
16 Erridge and Samani, 2009.
17 Huang et al., 2012.
18 Ijssennagger et al., 2015; Samraj et al., 2015.
19 For a detailed overview of the health risks associated with red meat chemicals, see Brown and Hazen (2015).
20 Koeth et al., 2013; Tang et al., 2013; Wang et al., 2011.
21 Demarquoy et al., 2004; Zeisel et al., 2003.
22 David et al., 2013.
23 For a detailed overview of the effects of gut bacteria on metabolism, see Nicholson et al. (2012), Sonnenburg and Bäckhed (2016), or Tremaroli and Bäckhed (2012).
24 Except for the treatment of *Clostridium difficile* infections (Gough et al., 2011).

25 Levy et al., 2015.
26 Vrieze et al., 2012.
27 Le Chatelier et al., 2013.
28 Tang et al., 2013.
29 Sun, 2012.
30 Chowdhury et al., 2014.
31 For a detailed overview of how fish fats decrease inflammation, see Fritsche (2015).
32 Oh et al., 2010.
33 Cao et al., 2008; Yore et al., 2014.
34 Caesar et al., 2015; Cintra et al., 2012; Lee et al., 2001; Oh et al., 2010; Shi et al., 2006.
35 Chowdhury et al., 2014.
36 For a detailed overview of the differences between animals and humans, see Nguyen et al. (2015), Seok et al. (2013) or Takao and Miyakawa (2015).
37 Fritsche, 2007.

Chapter 9

1 For a detailed overview of the health risks associated with sugar, see Lustig (2013) or Lustig (2014).
2 Di Luccia et al., 2015; Sellmann et al., 2015; Spruss et al., 2009, 2012.
3 A 32-ounce coke contains 86 grams of sugar (http://calorielab.com/restaurants/mcdonalds/coca-cola-classic-large/1/123), 60 per cent of which is likely to be fructose (Walker et al., 2014).
4 One raspberry has 0.04 grams of fructose (http://ndb.nal.usda.gov/ndb/foods/show/2374).
5 Teff et al., 2004.
6 Schoeller et al., 1997; Sinha et al., 1996.
7 Luo et al., 2015; Page et al., 2013.
8 For a detailed overview of the relationship between drinks and hunger, see Jones et al. (2014).
9 For a detailed overview of how the brain controls the release of insulin, ghrelin and other hormones, see Power and Schulkin (2008).
10 Crum et al., 2011.
11 Mattes, 2005; Tournier and Louis-Sylvestre, 1991.
12 Jones et al., 2014.
13 12 ounces of apple juice has about 140 calories and about 40 grams of sugar, while 12 ounces of coke has 140 calories and 39 grams of sugar (http://www.caloriecount.com/calories-apple-juice-i9400; http://www.caloriecount.com/calories-coca-cola-classic-i98047).
14 32 ounces of apple juice has about 108 grams of sugar, 50 per cent of which is fructose.
15 To get 32 ounces of juice requires about 1,800 grams of apples (http://www.vigopresses.co.uk/AdditionalDepartments/Header-Content/Make-apple-juice).
16 Walker et al., 2014.
17 For a detailed overview of alcohol metabolism, see Hawkins and Kalant (1972).
18 12 ounces of beer has about 150 calories (http://www.caloriecount.com/calories-beer-regular-i14003).
19 12 ounces of red wine has about 300 calories (http://www.caloriecount.com/calories-wine-table-red-i14096).
20 12 ounces of vodka has about 800 calories (http://www.caloriecount.com/calories-distilled-vodka-80-proof-i14051).
21 Suter and Tremblay, 2005.
22 Fernández-Solà, 2015.
23 For a detailed overview of the effects of alcohol on the body, see Krenz and Korthuis (2012).
24 In fact, coffee that is unfiltered (e.g. from a cafetière, or made in the "Turkish" style) does have a few calories. There are some fats in coffee beans that are transferred to the water when the coffee is brewed but they are removed by standard filtering. There is evidence from short-term human studies that these coffee fats can increase the production of liver fat packages (for an overview, see Cai et al., 2012) but there haven't yet been any studies of whether this increase persists in the long-term. And, strangely, these coffee fats don't seem to have any effect on the production of liver fat packages in animals (for an overview, see Urgert and Katan, 1997).

25 For a detailed overview of the effects of coffee on the body, see Rebello and van Dam (2013).
26 Freedman et al., 2012.
27 American Psychiatric Association, 2013.
28 Sturm and Hattori, 2013.
29 Merikangas and McClair, 2012.
30 Wang et al., 2001.
31 For a detailed overview of the role of dopamine in drug addiction, see Nutt et al. (2015).
32 Rada et al., 2005.
33 Avena et al., 2008.
34 Lenoir et al., 2007.

Chapter 10

1   Katz and Meller, 2014.
2   Alvaro et al., 2007.
3   Marette and Picard-Deland, 2014.
4   Hill et al., 1991.
5   Johnston et al., 2014.
6   Zeevi et al., 2015.
7   Carrots have a glycemic index of 32 and a glycemic load of 2 (http://www.health.harvard.edu/healthy-eating/glycemic_index_and_glycemic_load_for_100_foods).
8   Boiled spaghetti has a glycemic index of 58 and a glycemic load of 26 (http://www.health.harvard.edu/healthy-eating/glycemic_index_and_glycemic_load_for_100_foods).
9   For a detailed overview of the importance of protein, see Bilsborough and Mann (2006). For a detailed overview of the importance of vitamins and minerals, see Shenkin (2006b, 2006a).
10 Mattes and Donnelly, 1991.
11 O'Donnell et al., 2014; Stolarz-Skrzypek et al., 2011.
12 For a detailed overview of how kidneys regulate salt and how obesity disrupts kidney function, see Hall et al. (2012).
13 Hall et al. (2012).
14 For a detailed overview of the effects of high blood pressure on the heart, see Drazner (2011).
15 For a detailed overview of the effects of high blood pressure on blood vessels, see Johansson (1999) or Touyz (2004).
16 Mente et al., 2014.
17 Graudal et al., 1998; He and MacGregor, 2002.
18 He, J. et al., 1999; Tuomilehto et al., 2001.
19 Bjelakovic et al., 2013.
20 Moyer and U.S. Preventive Services Task Force (2014).
21 Rizos et al., 2012.
22 Chowdhury et al., 2014.
23 For a detailed overview of the potential health benefits of superfoods, see Del Rio et al. (2012).
24 For a detailed overview of the risks of deficiencies in vegetarian or vegan diets, see Craig (2010) or Key et al. (2006).
25 Micha et al., 2010; Siri-Tarino et al., 2010; de Souza et al., 2015; Sun, 2012.
26 Johnston et al., 2014.
27 For a detailed overview of the impact of meal timing on metabolism and health, see Mattson et al. (2014).

Chapter 11

1   For a detailed overview of the relationship between daily rhythms and metabolism, see Asher and Sassone-Corsi (2015) or Stenvers et al. (2012).
2   For a detailed overview of the brain clock, see Rosenwasser and Turek (2015).

3   For a detailed overview of what happens when daily rhythms break down, see Arble et al. (2010).
4   Hatori et al., 2012.
5   Feldmann et al., 2009.
6   For a detailed overview of gut bacteria rhythms, see Thaiss et al. (2015).
7   Leone et al., 2015; Mukherji et al., 2013.
8   For a detailed overview of the health risks associated with shift work, see Knutsson (2003).
9   Froy, 2012.
10 Dallmann et al., 2012; Morris et al., 2015; Scheer et al., 2009.
11 Gill and Panda, 2015.
12 For a detailed overview of the studies of disrupted daily rhythms in animals, see Arble et al. (2010).
13 Brandhorst et al., 2015.
14 For a detailed overview of the health benefits of taking long breaks from eating, see Longo and Mattson (2014) or Longo and Panda (2016).
15 Harvie et al., 2013, 2011.
16 Chaix et al., 2014.

Chapter 12

1   Jakubowicz et al., 2013.
2   Stote et al., 2007.
3   Bray et al., 2010.
4   Locke et al., 2015.
5   For a detailed overview of environmental influences on eating, see Wansink (2004) or Wansink and Chandon (2014).
6   Wansink et al., 2006.
7   For a comprehensive list of ways to avoid overeating, see Wansink (2014).
8   Dombrowski et al., 2014; Fildes et al., 2015; Kraschnewski et al., 2010; Mann et al., 2007.
9   Hall et al., 2011.
10 For a detailed overview of the metabolic changes that cause weight loss to slow down, see MacLean et al. (2011), Ochner et al. (2013) or Rosenbaum and Leibel (2010).
11 For a detailed overview of environmental influences on eating, see Wansink (2004) or Wansink and Chandon (2014).
12 Wing and Jeffery, 2001.
13 For a detailed overview of the effects of weight loss and regain on mental health, see Brownell and Rodin (1994).
14 Joyner and Green, 2009.
15 For a detailed overview of energy usage by muscles during exercise, see Egan and Zierath (2013).
16 Børsheim and Bahr, 2003.
17 For a detailed overview of the changes caused by exercise, see Egan and Zierath (2013) or Hawley et al. (2014).
18 For a detailed overview of the hormones released by muscles, see Pedersen and Febbraio (2012).
19 Ropelle et al., 2010.
20 Martins et al., 2008.
21 Starkie, 2003.
22 Willis et al., 2012.
23 Peake et al., 2005.
24 Aarts et al., 1997.
25 Urban et al., 2010, 2011.
26 Ravussin and Bogardus, 1989.
27 For a detailed overview of the difficulties involved in making calorie measurements, see Dulloo et al. (2012).

Glossary

If you want to learn more about anything, you can use this table to find the relevant scientific term.

Conversational term/phase	Scientific term/phrase
Glucose	
Stored glucose	Glycogen
Making glucose	Gluconeogenesis
Releasing glucose	Glycogenolysis
High/low blood glucose	Hyper/Hypoglycemia
Fat	
Stored fat	Triglyceride
Making fat	De novo lipogenesis
Releasing fat	Lipolysis
High/low blood fat	Hyper/Hypolipidemia or Hyper/Hypotriglyceridemia
Fat cell	Adipocyte
Body fat	Adipose tissue
Fat package	Lipoprotein
Digested fat package	Chylomicron
Liver fat package	Very-low-density lipoprotein (VLDL)
Waste package	High-density lipoprotein (HDL), "Good" cholesterol
Depleted digested fat package	Chylomicron remnant
Depleted liver fat package	Low-density lipoprotein (LDL), "Bad" cholesterol
Fat cell hormone	Adipokine
Fiber fats	Short-chain fatty acids (SCFAs)

Conversational term/phase	Scientific term/phrase
Fish fat	Omega-3 polyunsaturated fat
Belly fat	Visceral fat

Insulin

Insulin overshoot	Reactive postprandial hypoglycemia
High/low insulin	Hyper/Hypoinsulinemia
Pre-meal insulin release	Cephalic phase insulin response

Inflammation and disease

Build-up of waste	Oxidative stress
Waste	Reactive oxygen species (ROS)
Cells get overwhelmed	Endoplasmic reticulum (ER) stress
Immune cell chemical	Cytokine
Escort	Transporter
Cells get bigger and bigger	Hypertrophy
Cells don't get enough oxygen	Hypoxia
Build-up of plaques	Atherosclerosis
Bacterial pattern detector	Toll-like receptor
Fish fat pattern detector	GPR120
High blood pressure	Hypertension

Brain

Brain cell	Neuron
Pleasure system	Mesolimbic reward system
Self-control system	Dorsolateral prefrontal cortex
Stress system	Hypothalamic-pituitary-adrenal (HPA) axis
Cortisol	Glucocorticoids
Fidgeting	Non-exercise activity thermogenesis (NEAT)
Brain clock	Suprachiasmatic nucleus

Gut

Gut bacteria	Gut microbiota
Half-digested mush	Chyme

Conversational term/phase	Scientific term/phrase
Chemicals released by bacteria	Metabolites
Intestinal wall cells	Enterocytes
Ulcer bacteria	*Helicobacter pylori*
Bacteria-free mice	Germ-free or gnotobiotic mice
Bit of dead bacteria	Lipopolysaccharide (LPS)
Mucus bacteria	*Akkermansia muciniphila*

Other

Daily rhythms	Circadian rhythms
Red meat chemicals	Phosphatidylcholine, trimethylamine, trimethylamine-N-oxide
Muscle hormones	Myokines
Wasting energy by creating heat	(Diet-induced) thermogenesis

References

Aarts, H., Paulussen, T., and Schaalma, H. (1997). Physical exercise habit: on the conceptualization and formation of habitual health behaviours. Health Educ. Res. *12*, 363–374.

Abrams, G.D., Bauer, H., and Sprinz, H. (1963). Influence of the normal flora on mucosal morphology and cellular renewal in the ileum. A comparison of germ-free and conventional mice. Lab. Investig. J. Tech. Methods Pathol. *12*, 355–364.

Adam, T.C., and Epel, E.S. (2007). Stress, eating and the reward system. Physiol. Behav. *91*, 449–458.

Adiels, M., Olofsson, S.-O., Taskinen, M.-R., and Borén, J. (2008). Overproduction of very low–density lipoproteins is the hallmark of the dyslipidemia in the metabolic syndrome. Arterioscler. Thromb. Vasc. Biol. *28*, 1225–1236.

Alavanja, M.C.R., Hoppin, J.A., and Kamel, F. (2004). Health effects of chronic pesticide exposure: cancer and neurotoxicity. Annu. Rev. Public Health *25*, 155–197.

Alvaro, E., Andrieux, C., Rochet, V., Rigottier-Gois, L., Lepercq, P., Sutren, M., Galan, P., Duval, Y., Juste, C., and Doré, J. (2007). Composition and metabolism of the intestinal microbiota in consumers and non-consumers of yogurt. Br. J. Nutr. *97*, 126–133.

American Psychiatric Association (2013). Diagnostic and statistical manual of mental disorders: DSM-5 (American Psychiatric Publishing).

Arble, D.M., Ramsey, K.M., Bass, J., and Turek, F.W. (2010). Circadian disruption and metabolic disease: findings from animal models. Best Pract. Res. Clin. Endocrinol. Metab. *24*, 785–800.

Arnsten, A.F.T. (2015). Stress weakens prefrontal networks: molecular insults to higher cognition. Nat. Neurosci. *18*, 1376–1385.

Aron, A.R. (2007). The neural basis of inhibition in cognitive control. The Neuroscientist *13*, 214–228.

Arpaia, N., Campbell, C., Fan, X., Dikiy, S., van der Veeken, J., deRoos, P., Liu, H., Cross, J.R., Pfeffer, K., Coffer, P.J., et al. (2013). Metabolites produced by commensal bacteria promote peripheral regulatory T-cell generation. Nature *504*, 451–455.

Asher, G., and Sassone-Corsi, P. (2015). Time for food: the intimate interplay between nutrition, metabolism, and the circadian clock. Cell *161*, 84–92.

Aune, D., Keum, N., Giovannucci, E., Fadnes, L.T., Boffetta, P., Greenwood, D.C., Tonstad, S., Vatten, L.J., Riboli, E., and Norat, T. (2016). Whole grain consumption and risk of cardiovascular disease, cancer, and all-cause and cause-specific mortality: systematic review and dose-response meta-analysis of prospective studies. BMJ *353*, i2716.

Avena, N.M., Rada, P., and Hoebel, B.G. (2008). Evidence for sugar addiction: behavioral and neurochemical effects of intermittent, excessive sugar intake. Neurosci. Biobehav. Rev. *32*, 20–39.

Baicy, K., London, E.D., Monterosso, J., Wong, M.-L., Delibasi, T., Sharma, A., and Licinio, J. (2007). Leptin replacement alters brain response to food cues in genetically leptin-deficient adults. Proc. Natl. Acad. Sci. *104*, 18276–18279.

Barsh, G.S., Farooqi, I.S., and O'Rahilly, S. (2000). Genetics of body-weight regulation. Nature *404*, 644–651.

Bashir, M.E.H., Louie, S., Shi, H.N., and Nagler-Anderson, C. (2004). Toll-Like Receptor 4 signaling by intestinal microbes influences susceptibility to food allergy. J. Immunol. *172*, 6978–6987.

Bellentani, S., Scaglioni, F., Marino, M., and Bedogni, G. (2010). Epidemiology of non-alcoholic fatty liver disease. Dig. Dis. Basel Switz. *28*, 155–161.

Berger, S., Raman, G., Vishwanathan, R., Jacques, P.F., and Johnson, E.J. (2015). Dietary cholesterol and cardiovascular disease: a systematic review and meta-analysis. Am. J. Clin. Nutr. *102*, 276–294.

Berridge, K.C., and Kringelbach, M.L. (2015). Pleasure systems in the brain. Neuron *86*, 646–664.

Bersaglieri, T., Sabeti, P.C., Patterson, N., Vanderploeg, T., Schaffner, S.F., Drake, J.A., Rhodes, M., Reich, D.E., and Hirschhorn, J.N. (2004). Genetic signatures of strong recent positive selection at the lactase gene. Am. J. Hum. Genet. *74*, 1111–1120.

den Besten, G., van Eunen, K., Groen, A.K., Venema, K., Reijngoud, D.-J., and Bakker, B.M. (2013). The role of short-chain fatty acids in the interplay between diet, gut microbiota, and host energy metabolism. J. Lipid Res. *54*, 2325–2340.

Bilsborough, S., and Mann, N. (2006). A review of issues of dietary protein intake in humans. Int. J. Sport Nutr. Exerc. Metab. *16*, 129–152.

Bischoff, S.C., Barbara, G., Buurman, W., Ockhuizen, T., Schulzke, J.-D., Serino, M., Tilg, H., Watson, A., and Wells, J. (2014). Intestinal permeability – a new target for disease prevention and therapy. BMC Gastroenterol. *14*, 189.

Bjelakovic, G., Nikolova, D., and Gluud, C. (2013). Antioxidant supplements to prevent mortality. JAMA *310*, 1178–1179.

Björck, I., Granfeldt, Y., Liljeberg, H., Tovar, J., and Asp, N.G. (1994). Food properties affecting the digestion and absorption of carbohydrates. Am. J. Clin. Nutr. *59*, 699S–705S.

Blaser, M.J. (2014). Missing microbes: how the overuse of antibiotics is fueling our modern plagues (New York: Henry Holt and Company).

Boecker, H., Sprenger, T., Spilker, M.E., Henriksen, G., Koppenhoefer, M., Wagner, K.J., Valet, M., Berthele, A., and Tolle, T.R. (2008). The runner's high: opioidergic mechanisms in the human brain. Cereb. Cortex *18*, 2523–2531.

Børsheim, E., and Bahr, R. (2003). Effect of exercise intensity, duration and mode on post-exercise oxygen consumption. Sports Med. Auckl. NZ *33*, 1037–1060.

Bouchard, M.F., Bellinger, D.C., Wright, R.O., and Weisskopf, M.G. (2010). Attention-deficit/ hyperactivity disorder and urinary metabolites of organophosphate pesticides. Pediatrics *125*, e1270–e1277.

Brandhorst, S., Choi, I.Y., Wei, M., Cheng, C.W., Sedrakyan, S., Navarrete, G., Dubeau, L., Yap, L.P., Park, R., Vinciguerra, M., et al. (2015). A periodic diet that mimics fasting promotes multi-system regeneration, enhanced cognitive performance, and healthspan. Cell Metab. *22*, 86–99.

Bray, M.S., Tsai, J.-Y., Villegas-Montoya, C., Boland, B.B., Blasier, Z., Egbejimi, O., Kueht, M., and Young, M.E. (2010). Time-of-day-dependent dietary fat consumption influences multiple cardiometabolic syndrome parameters in mice. Int. J. Obes. *34*, 1589–1598.

Brookes, S.J.H., Spencer, N.J., Costa, M., and Zagorodnyuk, V.P. (2013). Extrinsic primary afferent signalling in the gut. Nat. Rev. Gastroenterol. Hepatol. *10*, 286–296.

Brown, J.M., and Hazen, S.L. (2015). The gut microbial endocrine organ: bacterially derived signals driving cardiometabolic diseases. Annu. Rev. Med. *66*, 343–359.

Brownell, K.D., and Rodin, J. (1994). Medical, metabolic, and psychological effects of weight cycling. Arch. Intern. Med. *154*, 1325–1330.

Bryan, N.S., Alexander, D.D., Coughlin, J.R., Milkowski, A.L., and Boffetta, P. (2012). Ingested nitrate and nitrite and stomach cancer risk: an updated review. Food Chem. Toxicol. *50*, 3646–3665.

Burrows, M.P., Volchkov, P., Kobayashi, K.S., and Chervonsky, A.V. (2015). Microbiota regulates type 1 diabetes through toll-like receptors. Proc. Natl. Acad. Sci. *112*, 9973–9977.

Butts, K.A., Weinberg, J., Young, A.H., and Phillips, A.G. (2011). Glucocorticoid receptors in the prefrontal cortex regulate stress-evoked dopamine efflux and aspects of executive function. Proc. Natl. Acad. Sci. U. S. A. *108*, 18459–18464.

Caesar, R., Tremaroli, V., Kovatcheva-Datchary, P., Cani, P.D., and Bäckhed, F. (2015). Crosstalk between gut microbiota and dietary lipids aggravates WAT inflammation through TLR signaling. Cell Metab. *22*, 658–668.

Cai, L., Ma, D., Zhang, Y., Liu, Z., and Wang, P. (2012). The effect of coffee consumption on serum lipids: a meta-analysis of randomized controlled trials. Eur. J. Clin. Nutr. *66*, 872–877.

Cani, P.D., Amar, J., Iglesias, M.A., Poggi, M., Knauf, C., Bastelica, D., Neyrinck, A.M., Fava, F., Tuohy, K.M., Chabo, C., et al. (2007). Metabolic endotoxemia initiates obesity and insulin resistance. Diabetes *56*, 1761–1772.

Cani, P.D., Bibiloni, R., Knauf, C., Waget, A., Neyrinck, A.M., Delzenne, N.M., and Burcelin, R. (2008). Changes in gut microbiota control metabolic endotoxemia-induced inflammation in high-fat diet-induced obesity and diabetes in mice. Diabetes *57*, 1470–1481.

Cao, H., Gerhold, K., Mayers, J.R., Wiest, M.M., Watkins, S.M., and Hotamisligil, G.S. (2008). Identification of a lipokine, a lipid hormone linking adipose tissue to systemic metabolism. Cell *134*, 933–944.

Chaix, A., Zarrinpar, A., Miu, P., and Panda, S. (2014). Time-restricted feeding is a preventative and therapeutic intervention against diverse nutritional challenges. Cell Metab. *20*, 991–1005.

Chassaing, B., Koren, O., Goodrich, J.K., Poole, A.C., Srinivasan, S., Ley, R.E., and Gewirtz, A.T. (2015). Dietary emulsifiers impact the mouse gut microbiota promoting colitis and metabolic syndrome. Nature *519*, 92–96.

Cho, I., Yamanishi, S., Cox, L., Methé, B.A., Zavadil, J., Li, K., Gao, Z., Mahana, D., Raju, K., Teitler, I., et al. (2012). Antibiotics in early life alter the murine colonic microbiome and adiposity. Nature *488*, 621–626.

Choi, S.H., and Ginsberg, H.N. (2011). Increased very low density lipoprotein (VLDL) secretion, hepatic steatosis, and insulin resistance. Trends Endocrinol. Metab. *22*, 353–363.

Chowdhury, R., Warnakula, S., Kunutsor, S., Crowe, F., Ward, H.A., Johnson, L., Franco, O.H. Butterworth, A.S., Forouhi, N.G., Thompson, S.G., et al. (2014). Association of dietary, circulating, and supplement fatty acids with coronary risk: a systematic review and meta-analysis. Ann. Intern. Med. *160*, 398–406.

Cintra, D.E., Ropelle, E.R., Moraes, J.C., Pauli, J.R., Morari, J., de Souza, C.T., Grimaldi, R., Stahl, M., Carvalheira, J.B., Saad, M.J., et al. (2012). Unsaturated fatty acids revert diet-induced hypothalamic inflammation in obesity. PLoS ONE *7*, e30571.

Clemente, J.C., Ursell, L.K., Parfrey, L.W., and Knight, R. (2012). The impact of the gut microbiota on human health: an integrative view. Cell *148*, 1258–1270.

Colborn, T. (2006). A case for revisiting the safety of pesticides: a closer look at neurodevelopment. Environ. Health Perspect. *114*, 10–17.

Collins, S.M., Surette, M., and Bercik, P. (2012). The interplay between the intestinal microbiota and the brain. Nat. Rev. Microbiol. *10*, 735–742.

Cota, D., Tschöp, M.H., Horvath, T.L., and Levine, A.S. (2006). Cannabinoids, opioids and eating behavior: The molecular face of hedonism? Brain Res. Rev. *51*, 85–107.

Cox, L.M., and Blaser, M.J. (2015). Antibiotics in early life and obesity. Nat. Rev. Endocrinol. *11*, 182–190.

Cox, L.M., Yamanishi, S., Sohn, J., Alekseyenko, A.V., Leung, J.M., Cho, I., Kim, S.G., Li, H., Gao, Z., Mahana, D., et al. (2014). Altering the intestinal microbiota during a critical developmental window has lasting metabolic consequences. Cell *158*, 705–721.

Craig, W.J. (2010). Nutrition concerns and health effects of vegetarian diets. Nutr. Clin. Pract. *25*, 613–620.

Cromwell, G.L. (2002). Why and how antibiotics are used in swine production. Anim. Biotechnol. *13*, 7–27.

Crum, A.J., Corbin, W.R., Brownell, K.D., and Salovey, P. (2011). Mind over milkshakes: mindsets, not just nutrients, determine ghrelin response. Health Psychol. *30*, 424–429.

Cryan, J.F., and Dinan, T.G. (2012). Mind-altering microorganisms: the impact of the gut microbiota on brain and behaviour. Nat. Rev. Neurosci. *13*, 701–712.

Dallman, M.F., Pecoraro, N., Akana, S.F., Fleur, S.E. la, Gomez, F., Houshyar, H., Bell, M.E., Bhatnagar, S., Laugero, K.D., and Manalo, S. (2003). Chronic stress and obesity: A new view of "comfort food." Proc. Natl. Acad. Sci. *100*, 11696–11701.

Dallmann, R., Viola, A.U., Tarokh, L., Cajochen, C., and Brown, S.A. (2012). The human circadian metabolome. Proc. Natl. Acad. Sci. *109*, 2625–2629.

Dangour, A.D., Lock, K., Hayter, A., Aikenhead, A., Allen, E., and Uauy, R. (2010). Nutrition-related health effects of organic foods: a systematic review. Am. J. Clin. Nutr. *92*, 203–210.

David, L.A., Maurice, C.F., Carmody, R.N., Gootenberg, D.B., Button, J.E., Wolfe, B.E., Ling, A.V., Devlin, A.S., Varma, Y., Fischbach, M.A., et al. (2013). Diet rapidly and reproducibly alters the human gut microbiome. Nature *505*, 559–563.

DeFrancesco, L. (2013). How safe does transgenic food need to be? Nat. Biotechnol. *31*, 794–802.

Del Rio, D., Rodriguez-Mateos, A., Spencer, J.P.E., Tognolini, M., Borges, G., and Crozier, A. (2012). Dietary (poly)phenolics in human health: structures, bioavailability, and evidence of protective effects against chronic diseases. Antioxid. Redox Signal. *18*, 1818–1892.

DelParigi, A., Chen, K., Salbe, A.D., Hill, J.O., Wing, R.R., Reiman, E.M., and Tataranni, P.A. (2006). Successful dieters have increased neural activity in cortical areas involved in the control of behavior. Int. J. Obes. *31*, 440–448.

Demarquoy, J., Georges, B., Rigault, C., Royer, M.-C., Clairet, A., Soty, M., Lekounoungou, S., and Le Borgne, F. (2004). Radioisotopic determination of L-carnitine content in foods commonly eaten in Western countries. Food Chem. *86*, 137–142.

Dethlefsen, L., and Relman, D.A. (2011). Incomplete recovery and individualized responses of the human distal gut microbiota to repeated antibiotic perturbation. Proc. Natl. Acad. Sci. *108*, 4554–4561.

Di Luccia, B., Crescenzo, R., Mazzoli, A., Cigliano, L., Venditti, P., Walser, J.-C., Widmer, A., Baccigalupi, L., Ricca, E., and Iossa, S. (2015). Rescue of fructose-induced metabolic syndrome by antibiotics or faecal transplantation in a rat model of obesity. PLOS ONE *10*, e0134893.

DiLeone, R.J., Taylor, J.R., and Picciotto, M.R. (2012). The drive to eat: comparisons and distinctions between mechanisms of food reward and drug addiction. Nat. Neurosci. *15*, 1330–1335.

Dombrowski, S.U., Knittle, K., Avenell, A., Araújo-Soares, V., and Sniehotta, F.F. (2014). Long term maintenance of weight loss with non-surgical interventions in obese adults: systematic review and meta-analyses of randomised controlled trials. BMJ *348*, g2646.

Donath, M.Y., and Shoelson, S.E. (2011). Type 2 diabetes as an inflammatory disease. Nat. Rev. Immunol. *11*, 98–107.

Drazner, M.H. (2011). The progression of hypertensive heart disease. Circulation *123*, 327–334.

Dulloo, A.G., Jacquet, J., Montani, J.-P., and Schutz, Y. (2012). Adaptive thermogenesis in human body weight regulation: more of a concept than a measurable entity?: Adaptive thermogenesis in humans. Obes. Rev. *13*, 105–121.

Duncan, R.E., Ahmadian, M., Jaworski, K., Sarkadi-Nagy, E., and Sul, H.S. (2007). Regulation of lipolysis in adipocytes. Annu. Rev. Nutr. *27*, 79–101.

Egan, B., and Zierath, J.R. (2013). Exercise metabolism and the molecular regulation of skeletal muscle adaptation. Cell Metab. *17*, 162–184.

Elinav, E., Strowig, T., Kau, A.L., Henao-Mejia, J., Thaiss, C.A., Booth, C.J., Peaper, D.R., Bertin, J., Eisenbarth, S.C., Gordon, J.I., et al. (2011). NLRP6 inflammasome regulates colonic microbial ecology and risk for colitis. Cell *145*, 745–757.

Emmons, K.M., Marcus, B.H., Linnan, L., Rossi, J.S., and Abrams, D.B. (1994). Mechanisms in multiple risk factor interventions: smoking, physical activity, and dietary fat intake among manufacturing workers. Prev. Med. *23*, 481–489.

Erridge, C., and Samani, N.J. (2009). Saturated fatty acids do not directly stimulate toll-like receptor signaling. Arterioscler. Thromb. Vasc. Biol. *29*, 1944–1949.

Everard, A., Belzer, C., Geurts, L., Ouwerkerk, J.P., Druart, C., Bindels, L.B., Guiot, Y., Derrien, M., Muccioli, G.G., Delzenne, N.M., et al. (2013). Cross-talk between Akkermansia muciniphila and intestinal epithelium controls diet-induced obesity. Proc. Natl. Acad. Sci. *110*, 9066–9071.

Feldmann, H.M., Golozoubova, V., Cannon, B., and Nedergaard, J. (2009). UCP1 ablation induces obesity and abolishes diet-induced thermogenesis in mice exempt from thermal stress by living at thermoneutrality. Cell Metab. *9*, 203–209.

Fernandes, M.F.A., Matthys, D., Hryhorczuk, C., Sharma, S., Mogra, S., Alquier, T., and Fulton, S. (2015). Leptin suppresses the rewarding effects of running via stat3 signaling in dopamine neurons. Cell Metab. *22*, 741–749.

Fernández-Solà, J. (2015). Cardiovascular risks and benefits of moderate and heavy alcohol consumption. Nat. Rev. Cardiol. *12*, 576–587.

Fildes, A., Charlton, J., Rudisill, C., Littlejohns, P., Prevost, A.T., and Gulliford, M.C. (2015). Probability of an obese person attaining normal body weight: cohort study using electronic health records. Am. J. Public Health *105*, e54-59.

Freedman, N.D., Park, Y., Abnet, C.C., Hollenbeck, A.R., and Sinha, R. (2012). Association of coffee drinking with total and cause-specific mortality. N. Engl. J. Med. *366*, 1891–1904.

Fritsche, K. (2007). Important differences exist in the dose-response relationship between diet and immune cell fatty acids in humans and rodents. Lipids *42*, 961–979.

Fritsche, K.L. (2015). The science of fatty acids and inflammation. Adv. Nutr. Int. Rev. J. *6*, 293S–301S.

Froy, O. (2012). Circadian rhythms and obesity in mammals. ISRN Obes. *2012*, 1–12.

Garber, A.K., and Lustig, R.H. (2011). Is fast food addictive? Curr. Drug Abuse Rev. *4*, 146–162.

Garland, T., Schutz, H., Chappell, M.A., Keeney, B.K., Meek, T.H., Copes, L.E., Acosta, W., Drenowatz, C., Maciel, R.C., van Dijk, G., et al. (2011). The biological control of voluntary exercise, spontaneous physical activity and daily energy expenditure in relation to obesity: human and rodent perspectives. J. Exp. Biol. *214*, 206–229.

Garrett, W.S., Gordon, J.I., and Glimcher, L.H. (2010). Homeostasis and inflammation in the intestine. Cell *140*, 859–870.

Ghoshal, S., Witta, J., Zhong, J., de Villiers, W., and Eckhardt, E. (2008). Chylomicrons promote intestinal absorption of lipopolysaccharides. J. Lipid Res. *50*, 90–97.

Gil-Campos, M., Aguilera, C.M., Cañete, R., and Gil, A. (2006). Ghrelin: a hormone regulating food intake and energy homeostasis. Br. J. Nutr. *96*, 201.

Gilden, R.C., Huffling, K., and Sattler, B. (2010). Pesticides and health risks. J. Obstet. Gynecol. Neonatal Nurs. *39*, 103–110.

Gill, S., and Panda, S. (2015). A smartphone app reveals erratic diurnal eating patterns in humans that can be modulated for health benefits. Cell Metab. *22*, 789–798.

Gleeson, M., Bishop, N.C., Stensel, D.J., Lindley, M.R., Mastana, S.S., and Nimmo, M.A. (2011). The anti-inflammatory effects of exercise: mechanisms and implications for the prevention and treatment of disease. Nat. Rev. Immunol. *11*, 607–615.

Glimcher, P.W. (2011). Understanding dopamine and reinforcement learning: the dopamine reward prediction error hypothesis. Proc. Natl. Acad. Sci. U. S. A. *108 Suppl 3*, 15647–15654.

Goodrich, J.K., Waters, J.L., Poole, A.C., Sutter, J.L., Koren, O., Blekhman, R., Beaumont, M., Van Treuren, W., Knight, R., Bell, J.T., et al. (2014). Human genetics shape the gut microbiome. Cell *159*, 789–799.

Gough, E., Shaikh, H., and Manges, A.R. (2011). Systematic review of intestinal microbiota transplantation (fecal bacteriotherapy) for recurrent clostridium difficile infection. Clin. Infect. Dis. *53*, 994–1002.

Graudal, N.A., Galløe, A.M., and Garred, P. (1998). Effects of sodium restriction on blood pressure, renin, aldosterone, catecholamines, cholesterols, and triglyceride: a meta-analysis. JAMA *279*, 1383–1391.

Gregor, M.F., and Hotamisligil, G.S. (2011). Inflammatory mechanisms in obesity. Annu. Rev. Immunol. *29*, 415–445.

Guo, J., Simmons, W.K., Herscovitch, P., Martin, A., and Hall, K.D. (2014). Striatal dopamine D2-like receptor correlation patterns with human obesity and opportunistic eating behavior. Mol. Psychiatry *19*, 1078–1084.

Hall, J.E., Granger, J.P., do Carmo, J.M., da Silva, A.A., Dubinion, J., George, E., Hamza, S., Speed, J., and Hall, M.E. (2012). Hypertension: physiology and pathophysiology. In Comprehensive Physiology, R. Terjung, ed. (Hoboken, NJ, USA: John Wiley & Sons, Inc.)

Hall, K.D., Sacks, G., Chandramohan, D., Chow, C.C., Wang, Y.C., Gortmaker, S.L., and Swinburn, B.A. (2011). Quantification of the effect of energy imbalance on bodyweight. The Lancet *378*, 826–837.

Harvie, M., Wright, C., Pegington, M., McMullan, D., Mitchell, E., Martin, B., Cutler, R.G., Evans, G., Whiteside, S., Maudsley, S., et al. (2013). The effect of intermittent energy and carbohydrate restriction v. daily energy restriction on weight loss and metabolic disease risk markers in overweight women. Br. J. Nutr. *110*, 1534–1547.

Harvie, M.N., Pegington, M., Mattson, M.P., Frystyk, J., Dillon, B., Evans, G., Cuzick, J., Jebb, S.A., Martin, B., Cutler, R.G., et al. (2011). The effects of intermittent or continuous energy restriction on weight loss and metabolic disease risk markers: a randomized trial in young overweight women. Int. J. Obes. 2005 *35*, 714–727.

Hatori, M., Vollmers, C., Zarrinpar, A., DiTacchio, L., Bushong, E.A., Gill, S., Leblanc, M., Chaix, A., Joens, M., Fitzpatrick, J.A.J., et al. (2012). Time-restricted feeding without reducing caloric intake prevents metabolic diseases in mice fed a high-fat diet. Cell Metab. *15*, 848–860.

Hawkins, R.D., and Kalant, H. (1972). The metabolism of ethanol and its metabolic effects. Pharmacol. Rev. *24*, 67–157.

Hawley, J.A., Hargreaves, M., Joyner, M.J., and Zierath, J.R. (2014). Integrative biology of exercise. Cell *159*, 738–749.

He, F.J., and MacGregor, G.A. (2002). Effect of modest salt reduction on blood pressure: a meta-analysis of randomized trials. Implications for public health. J. Hum. Hypertens. *16*, 761–770.

He, J., Ogden, L.G., Vupputuri, S., Bazzano, L.A., Loria, C., and Whelton, P.K. (1999). Dietary sodium intake and subsequent risk of cardiovascular disease in overweight adults. JAMA *282*, 2027–2034.

Hecht, S.S. (1999). Tobacco smoke carcinogens and lung cancer. J. Natl. Cancer Inst. *91*, 1194–1210.

Henao-Mejia, J., Elinav, E., Jin, C., Hao, L., Mehal, W.Z., Strowig, T., Thaiss, C.A., Kau, A.L., Eisenbarth, S.C., Jurczak, M.J., et al. (2012). Inflammasome-mediated dysbiosis regulates progression of NAFLD and obesity. Nature 482, 179–185.

Hill, D.A., Siracusa, M.C., Abt, M.C., Kim, B.S., Kobuley, D., Kubo, M., Kambayashi, T., LaRosa, D.F., Renner, E.D., Orange, J.S., et al. (2012). Commensal bacteria–derived signals regulate basophil hematopoiesis and allergic inflammation. Nat. Med. 18, 538–546.

Hill, J.O., Peters, J.C., Reed, G.W., Schlundt, D.G., Sharp, T., and Greene, H.L. (1991). Nutrient balance in humans: effects of diet composition. Am. J. Clin. Nutr. 54, 10–17.

Hommel, J.D., Trinko, R., Sears, R.M., Georgescu, D., Liu, Z.-W., Gao, X.-B., Thurmon, J.J., Marinelli, M., and DiLeone, R.J. (2006). Leptin receptor signaling in midbrain dopamine neurons regulates feeding. Neuron 51, 801–810.

Hooper, L.V., Littman, D.R., and Macpherson, A.J. (2012). Interactions between the microbiota and the immune system. Science 336, 1268–1273.

Hotamisligil, G.S. (2010). Endoplasmic reticulum stress and the inflammatory basis of metabolic disease. Cell 140, 900–917.

Huang, S., Rutkowsky, J.M., Snodgrass, R.G., Ono-Moore, K.D., Schneider, D.A., Newman, J.W., Adams, S.H., and Hwang, D.H. (2012). Saturated fatty acids activate TLR-mediated proinflammatory signaling pathways. J. Lipid Res. 53, 2002–2013.

Ibrahim, M.M. (2010). Subcutaneous and visceral adipose tissue: structural and functional differences. Obes. Rev. Off. J. Int. Assoc. Study Obes. 11, 11–18.

Ijssennagger, N., Belzer, C., Hooiveld, G.J., Dekker, J., van Mil, S.W.C., Müller, M., Kleerebezem, M., and van der Meer, R. (2015). Gut microbiota facilitates dietary heme-induced epithelial hyperproliferation by opening the mucus barrier in colon. Proc. Natl. Acad. Sci. 112, 10038–10043.

Inzlicht, M., Schmeichel, B.J., and Macrae, C.N. (2014). Why self-control seems (but may not be) limited. Trends Cogn. Sci. 18, 127–133.

Jakubowicz, D., Barnea, M., Wainstein, J., and Froy, O. (2013). High caloric intake at breakfast vs. dinner differentially influences weight loss of overweight and obese women: effect of high-calorie breakfast vs. dinner. Obesity 21, 2504–2512.

Jha, P. (2009). Avoidable global cancer deaths and total deaths from smoking. Nat. Rev. Cancer 9, 655–664.

Johansson, B.B. (1999). Hypertension mechanisms causing stroke. Clin. Exp. Pharmacol. Physiol. 26, 563–565.

Johnston, B.C., Kanters, S., Bandayrel, K., Wu, P., Naji, F., Siemieniuk, R.A., Ball, G.D.C., Busse, J.W., Thorlund, K., Guyatt, G., et al. (2014). Comparison of weight loss among named diet programs in overweight and obese adults: a meta-analysis. JAMA 312, 923.

Jones, J.B., Lee, J., and Mattes, R.D. (2014). Solid versus liquid calories: current scientific understandings. In Fructose, high fructose corn syrup, sucrose and health, J.M. Rippe, ed. (New York, NY: Springer New York).

Joyner, M.J., and Green, D.J. (2009). Exercise protects the cardiovascular system: effects beyond traditional risk factors. J. Physiol. 587, 5551–5558.

Kaprio, J., Tuomilehto, J., Koskenvuo, M., Romanov, K., Reunanen, A., Eriksson, J., Stengård, J., and Kesäniemi, Y.A. (1992). Concordance for type 1 (insulin-dependent) and type 2 (non-insulin-dependent) diabetes mellitus in a population-based cohort of twins in Finland. Diabetologia 35, 1060–1067.

Karlsson, H.K., Tuominen, L., Tuulari, J.J., Hirvonen, J., Parkkola, R., Helin, S., Salminen, P., Nuutila, P., and Nummenmaa, L. (2015). Obesity is associated with decreased opioid but unaltered dopamine d2 receptor availability in the brain. J. Neurosci. 35, 3959–3965.

Katz, D.L., and Meller, S. (2014). Can we say what diet is best for health? Annu. Rev. Public Health 35, 83–103.

Kenny, P.J. (2011). Reward mechanisms in obesity: new insights and future directions. Neuron 69, 664–679.

Key, T.J., Appleby, P.N., and Rosell, M.S. (2006). Health effects of vegetarian and vegan diets. Proc. Nutr. Soc. 65, 35–41.

Klümper, W., and Qaim, M. (2014). A meta-analysis of the impacts of genetically modified crops. PLoS ONE 9, e111629.

Knip, M., and Siljander, H. (2016). The role of the intestinal microbiota in type 1 diabetes mellitus. Nat. Rev. Endocrinol. Advance online publication.

Knutsson, A. (2003). Health disorders of shift workers. Occup. Med. Oxf. Engl. 53, 103–108.

Koeth, R.A., Wang, Z., Levison, B.S., Buffa, J.A., Org, E., Sheehy, B.T., Britt, E.B., Fu, X., Wu, Y., Li, L., et al. (2013). Intestinal microbiota metabolism of L-carnitine, a nutrient in red meat, promotes atherosclerosis. Nat. Med. *19*, 576–585.

Kohno, D., Gao, H.-Z., Muroya, S., Kikuyama, S., and Yada, T. (2003). Ghrelin directly interacts with neuropeptide-Y-containing neurons in the rat arcuate nucleus: Ca2+ signaling via protein kinase A and N-type channel-dependent mechanisms and cross-talk with leptin and orexin. Diabetes *52*, 948–956.

Kotz, C.M., Teske, J.A., and Billington, C.J. (2008). Neuroregulation of nonexercise activity thermogenesis and obesity resistance. AJP Regul. Integr. Comp. Physiol. *294*, R699–R710.

Kraschnewski, J.L., Boan, J., Esposito, J., Sherwood, N.E., Lehman, E.B., Kephart, D.K., and Sciamanna, C.N. (2010). Long-term weight loss maintenance in the United States. Int. J. Obes. *34*, 1644–1654.

Krenz, M., and Korthuis, R.J. (2012). Moderate ethanol ingestion and cardiovascular protection: from epidemiologic associations to cellular mechanisms. J. Mol. Cell. Cardiol. *52*, 93–104.

Lancaster, G.I., and Febbraio, M.A. (2014). The immunomodulating role of exercise in metabolic disease. Trends Immunol. *35*, 262–269.

Laugerette, F., Vors, C., Géloën, A., Chauvin, M.-A., Soulage, C., Lambert-Porcheron, S., Peretti, N., Alligier, M., Burcelin, R., Laville, M., et al. (2011). Emulsified lipids increase endotoxemia: possible role in early postprandial low-grade inflammation. J. Nutr. Biochem. *22*, 53–59.

Laxminarayan, R., Duse, A., Wattal, C., Zaidi, A.K.M., Wertheim, H.F.L., Sumpradit, N., Vlieghe, E., Hara, G.L., Gould, I.M., Goossens, H., et al. (2013). Antibiotic resistance—the need for global solutions. Lancet Infect. Dis. *13*, 1057–1098.

Lazo, M., Hernaez, R., Eberhardt, M.S., Bonekamp, S., Kamel, I., Guallar, E., Koteish, A., Brancati, F.L., and Clark, J.M. (2013). Prevalence of nonalcoholic fatty liver disease in the United States: the Third National Health and Nutrition Examination Survey, 1988–1994. Am. J. Epidemiol. *178*, 38–45.

Le Chatelier, E., Nielsen, T., Qin, J., Prifti, E., Hildebrand, F., Falony, G., Almeida, M., Arumugam, M., Batto, J.-M., Kennedy, S., et al. (2013). Richness of human gut microbiome correlates with metabolic markers. Nature *500*, 541–546.

Le Merrer, J., Becker, J.A.J., Befort, K., and Kieffer, B.L. (2009). Reward processing by the opioid system in the brain. Physiol. Rev. *89*, 1379–1412.

LeBlanc, J.G., Milani, C., de Giori, G.S., Sesma, F., van Sinderen, D., and Ventura, M. (2013). Bacteria as vitamin suppliers to their host: a gut microbiota perspective. Curr. Opin. Biotechnol. *24*, 160–168.

Lee, Y.K., and Mazmanian, S.K. (2010). Has the microbiota played a critical role in the evolution of the adaptive immune system? Science *330*, 1768–1773.

Lee, J.Y., Sohn, K.H., Rhee, S.H., and Hwang, D. (2001). Saturated fatty acids, but not unsaturated fatty acids, induce the expression of cyclooxygenase-2 mediated through toll-like receptor 4. J. Biol. Chem. *276*, 16683–16689.

Lenoir, M., Serre, F., Cantin, L., and Ahmed, S.H. (2007). Intense sweetness surpasses cocaine reward. PloS One *2*, e698.

Leone, V., Gibbons, S.M., Martinez, K., Hutchison, A.L., Huang, E.Y., Cham, C.M., Pierre, J.F., Heneghan, A.F., Nadimpalli, A., Hubert, N., et al. (2015). Effects of diurnal variation of gut microbes and high-fat feeding on host circadian clock function and metabolism. Cell Host Microbe *17*, 681–689.

Levine, J.A., Eberhardt, N.L., and Jensen, M.D. (1999). Role of nonexercise activity thermogenesis in resistance to fat gain in humans. Science *283*, 212–214.

Levine, J.A., Lanningham-Foster, L.M., McCrady, S.K., Krizan, A.C., Olson, L.R., Kane, P.H., Jensen, M.D., and Clark, M.M. (2005). Interindividual variation in posture allocation: possible role in human obesity. Science *307*, 584–586.

Levy, M., Thaiss, C.A., Zeevi, D., Dohnalová, L., Zilberman-Schapira, G., Mahdi, J.A., David, E., Savidor, A., Korem, T., Herzig, Y., et al. (2015). Microbiota-modulated metabolites shape the intestinal microenvironment by regulating NLRP6 inflammasome signaling. Cell *163*, 1428–1443.

Ley, R.E., Hamady, M., Lozupone, C., Turnbaugh, P.J., Ramey, R.R., Bircher, J.S., Schlegel, M.L., Tucker, T.A., Schrenzel, M.D., Knight, R., et al. (2008). Evolution of mammals and their gut microbes. Science *320*, 1647–1651.

Liesa, M., and Shirihai, O.S. (2013). Mitochondrial dynamics in the regulation of nutrient utilization and energy expenditure. Cell Metab. *17*, 491–506.

Livesey, G., and Elia, M. (1988). Estimation of energy expenditure, net carbohydrate utilization, and net fat oxidation and synthesis by indirect calorimetry: evaluation of errors with special reference to the detailed composition of fuels. Am. J. Clin. Nutr. *47*, 608–628.

Locke, A.E., Kahali, B., Berndt, S.I., Justice, A.E., Pers, T.H., Day, F.R., Powell, C., Vedantam, S., Buchkovich, M.L., Yang, J., et al. (2015). Genetic studies of body mass index yield new insights for obesity biology. Nature *518*, 197–206.

Longo, V.D., and Mattson, M.P. (2014). Fasting: molecular mechanisms and clinical applications. Cell Metab. *19*, 181–192.

Longo, V.D., and Panda, S. (2016). Fasting, circadian rhythms, and time-restricted feeding in healthy lifespan. Cell Metab. *23*, 1048–1059.

Lopez-Garcia, E., Schulze, M.B., Meigs, J.B., Manson, J.E., Rifai, N., Stampfer, M.J., Willett, W.C., and Hu, F.B. (2005). Consumption of trans fatty acids is related to plasma biomarkers of inflammation and endothelial dysfunction. J. Nutr. *135*, 562–566.

Lozupone, C.A., Stombaugh, J.I., Gordon, J.I., Jansson, J.K., and Knight, R. (2012). Diversity, stability and resilience of the human gut microbiota. Nature *489*, 220–230.

Ludwig, D.S., Majzoub, J.A., Al-Zahrani, A., Dallal, G.E., Blanco, I., and Roberts, S.B. (1999). High glycemic index foods, overeating, and obesity. Pediatrics *103*, E26.

Lumeng, C.N., Bodzin, J.L., and Saltiel, A.R. (2007). Obesity induces a phenotypic switch in adipose tissue macrophage polarization. J. Clin. Invest. *117*, 175–184.

Luo, S., Monterosso, J.R., Sarpelleh, K., and Page, K.A. (2015). Differential effects of fructose versus glucose on brain and appetitive responses to food cues and decisions for food rewards. Proc. Natl. Acad. Sci. *112*, 6509–6514.

Lustig, D.R. (2014). Fat chance: the hidden truth about sugar, obesity and disease (London: Fourth Estate).

Lustig, R.H. (2013). Fructose: it's "alcohol without the buzz." Adv. Nutr. Int. Rev. J. *4*, 226–235.

MacLean, P.S., Bergouignan, A., Cornier, M.-A., and Jackman, M.R. (2011). Biology's response to dieting: the impetus for weight regain. AJP Regul. Integr. Comp. Physiol. *301*, R581–R600.

Major, G.C., Doucet, E., Trayhurn, P., Astrup, A., and Tremblay, A. (2007). Clinical significance of adaptive thermogenesis. Int. J. Obes. *31*, 204–212.

Manichanh, C., Borruel, N., Casellas, F., and Guarner, F. (2012). The gut microbiota in IBD. Nat. Rev. Gastroenterol. Hepatol. *9*, 599–608.

Mann, T., Tomiyama, A.J., Westling, E., Lew, A.-M., Samuels, B., and Chatman, J. (2007). Medicare's search for effective obesity treatments: diets are not the answer. Am. Psychol. *62*, 220–233.

Marette, A., and Picard-Deland, E. (2014). Yogurt consumption and impact on health: focus on children and cardiometabolic risk. Am. J. Clin. Nutr. *99*, 1243S–1247S.

Martins, C., Morgan, L., and Truby, H. (2008). A review of the effects of exercise on appetite regulation: an obesity perspective. Int. J. Obes. 2005 *32*, 1337–1347.

Maslowski, K.M., Vieira, A.T., Ng, A., Kranich, J., Sierro, F., Di, Y., Schilter, H.C., Rolph, M.S., Mackay, F., Artis, D., et al. (2009). Regulation of inflammatory responses by gut microbiota and chemoattractant receptor GPR43. Nature *461*, 1282–1286.

Massadi, O., Lear, P., Muller, T., Lopez, M., Dieguez, C., Tschop, M., and Nogueiras, R. (2014). Review of novel aspects of the regulation of ghrelin secretion. Curr. Drug Metab. *15*, 398–413.

Mattes, R. (2005). Soup and satiety. Physiol. Behav. *83*, 739–747.

Mattes, R.D., and Donnelly, D. (1991). Relative contributions of dietary sodium sources. J. Am. Coll. Nutr. *10*, 383–393.

Mattson, M.P., Allison, D.B., Fontana, L., Harvie, M., Longo, V.D., Malaisse, W.J., Mosley, M., Notterpek, L., Ravussin, E., Scheer, F.A.J.L., et al. (2014). Meal frequency and timing in health and disease. Proc. Natl. Acad. Sci. *111*, 16647–16653.

Mauger, J.-F., Lichtenstein, A.H., Ausman, L.M., Jalbert, S.M., Jauhiainen, M., Ehnholm, C., and Lamarche, B. (2003). Effect of different forms of dietary hydrogenated fats on LDL particle size. Am. J. Clin. Nutr. *78*, 370–375.

Mazmanian, S.K., Liu, C.H., Tzianabos, A.O., and Kasper, D.L. (2005). An immunomodulatory molecule of symbiotic bacteria directs maturation of the host immune system. Cell *122*, 107–118.

McCue, M.D. (2010). Starvation physiology: reviewing the different strategies animals use to survive a common challenge. Comp. Biochem. Physiol. A. Mol. Integr. Physiol. *156*, 1–18.

McEwen, B.S., Bowles, N.P., Gray, J.D., Hill, M.N., Hunter, R.G., Karatsoreos, I.N., and Nasca, C. (2015). Mechanisms of stress in the brain. Nat. Neurosci. *18*, 1353–1363.

Mente, A., O'Donnell, M.J., Rangarajan, S., McQueen, M.J., Poirier, P., Wielgosz, A., Morrison, H., Li, W., Wang, X., Di, C., et al. (2014). Association of urinary sodium and potassium excretion with blood pressure. N. Engl. J. Med. *371*, 601–611.

Merikangas, K.R., and McClair, V.L. (2012). Epidemiology of substance use disorders. Hum. Genet. *131*, 779–789.

Micha, R., Wallace, S.K., and Mozaffarian, D. (2010). Red and processed meat consumption and risk of incident coronary heart disease, stroke, and diabetes mellitus: a systematic review and meta-analysis. Circulation *121*, 2271–2283.

Mikkelsen, K.H., Knop, F.K., Frost, M., Hallas, J., and Pottegård, A. (2015). Use of antibiotics and risk of type 2 diabetes: a population-based case-control study. J. Clin. Endocrinol. Metab. *100*, 3633–3640.

Milanski, M., Degasperi, G., Coope, A., Morari, J., Denis, R., Cintra, D.E., Tsukumo, D.M.L., Anhe, G., Amaral, M.E., Takahashi, H.K., et al. (2009). Saturated fatty acids produce an inflammatory response predominantly through the activation of tlr4 signaling in hypothalamus: implications for the pathogenesis of obesity. J. Neurosci. *29*, 359–370.

Miller, G.E., Chen, E., Sze, J., Marin, T., Arevalo, J.M.G., Doll, R., Ma, R., and Cole, S.W. (2008). A functional genomic fingerprint of chronic stress in humans: blunted glucocorticoid and increased NF-κB signaling. Biol. Psychiatry *64*, 266–272.

Morris, C.J., Yang, J.N., Garcia, J.I., Myers, S., Bozzi, I., Wang, W., Buxton, O.M., Shea, S.A., and Scheer, F.A.J.L. (2015). Endogenous circadian system and circadian misalignment impact glucose tolerance via separate mechanisms in humans. Proc. Natl. Acad. Sci. *112*, E2225–E2234.

Morton, A.M., Sefik, E., Upadhyay, R., Weissleder, R., Benoist, C., and Mathis, D. (2014). Endoscopic photoconversion reveals unexpectedly broad leukocyte trafficking to and from the gut. Proc. Natl. Acad. Sci. U. S. A. *111*, 6696–6701.

Morton, G.J., Kaiyala, K.J., Fisher, J.D., Ogimoto, K., Schwartz, M.W., and Wisse, B.E. (2011). Identification of a physiological role for leptin in the regulation of ambulatory activity and wheel running in mice. AJP Endocrinol. Metab. *300*, E392–E401.

Moyer, V.A., and U.S. Preventive Services Task Force. (2014). Vitamin, mineral, and multivitamin supplements for the primary prevention of cardiovascular disease and cancer: U.S. Preventive Services Task Force recommendation statement. Ann. Intern. Med. *160*, 558–564.

Mozaffarian, D., Pischon, T., Hankinson, S.E., Rifai, N., Joshipura, K., Willett, W.C., and Rimm, E.B. (2004). Dietary intake of trans fatty acids and systemic inflammation in women. Am. J. Clin. Nutr. *79*, 606–612.

Mozaffarian, D., Katan, M.B., Ascherio, A., Stampfer, M.J., and Willett, W.C. (2006). Trans fatty acids and cardiovascular disease. N. Engl. J. Med. *354*, 1601–1613.

Mukherji, A., Kobiita, A., Ye, T., and Chambon, P. (2013). Homeostasis in intestinal epithelium is orchestrated by the circadian clock and microbiota cues transduced by TLRs. Cell *153*, 812–827.

Musunuru, K. (2010). Atherogenic dyslipidemia: cardiovascular risk and dietary intervention. Lipids *45*, 907–914.

Myers, M.G. (2015). Leptin keeps working, even in obesity. Cell Metab. *21*, 791–792.

Myers, M.G., Heymsfield, S.B., Haft, C., Kahn, B.B., Laughlin, M., Leibel, R.L., Tschöp, M.H., and Yanovski, J.A. (2012). Challenges and opportunities of defining clinical leptin resistance. Cell Metab. *15*, 150–156.

Neltner, T.G., Alger, H.M., O'Reilly, J.T., Krimsky, S., Bero, L.A., and Maffini, M.V. (2013). Conflicts of interest in approvals of additives to food determined to be generally recognized as safe: out of balance. JAMA Intern. Med. *173*, 2032–2036.

Ng, M., Fleming, T., Robinson, M., Thomson, B., Graetz, N., Margono, C., Mullany, E.C., Biryukov, S., Abbafati, C., Abera, S.F., et al. (2014). Global, regional, and national prevalence of overweight and obesity in children and adults during 1980–2013: a systematic analysis for the Global Burden of Disease Study 2013. The Lancet *384*, 766–781.

Nguyen, T.L.A., Vieira-Silva, S., Liston, A., and Raes, J. (2015). How informative is the mouse for human gut microbiota research? Dis. Model. Mech. *8*, 1–16.

Nicholson, J.K., Holmes, E., Kinross, J., Burcelin, R., Gibson, G., Jia, W., and Pettersson, S. (2012). Host-gut microbiota metabolic interactions. Science *336*, 1262–1267.

Nielsen, S., Guo, Z., Johnson, C.M., Hensrud, D.D., and Jensen, M.D. (2004). Splanchnic lipolysis in human obesity. J. Clin. Invest. *113*, 1582–1588.

Nutt, D.J., Lingford-Hughes, A., Erritzoe, D., and Stokes, P.R.A. (2015). The dopamine theory of addiction: 40 years of highs and lows. Nat. Rev. Neurosci. *16*, 305–312.

Nwokolo, C.U., Freshwater, D.A., O'Hare, P., and Randeva, H.S. (2003). Plasma ghrelin following cure of Helicobacter pylori. Gut *52*, 637–640.

Ochner, C.N., Barrios, D.M., Lee, C.D., and Pi-Sunyer, F.X. (2013). Biological mechanisms that promote weight regain following weight loss in obese humans. Physiol. Behav. *120*, 106–113.

O'Connor, E.C., Kremer, Y., Lefort, S., Harada, M., Pascoli, V., Rohner, C., and Lüscher, C. (2015). Accumbal D1R neurons projecting to lateral hypothalamus authorize feeding. Neuron *88*, 553–564.

Odegaard, J.I., and Chawla, A. (2013). Pleiotropic actions of insulin resistance and inflammation in metabolic homeostasis. Science *339*, 172–177.

O'Donnell, M., Mente, A., Rangarajan, S., McQueen, M.J., Wang, X., Liu, L., Yan, H., Lee, S.F., Mony, P., Devanath, A., et al. (2014). Urinary sodium and potassium excretion, mortality, and cardiovascular events. N. Engl. J. Med. *371*, 612–623.

Oh, D.Y., Talukdar, S., Bae, E.J., Imamura, T., Morinaga, H., Fan, W., Li, P., Lu, W.J., Watkins, S.M., and Olefsky, J.M. (2010). GPR120 is an omega-3 fatty acid receptor mediating potent anti-inflammatory and insulin-sensitizing effects. Cell *142*, 687–698.

Oldroyd, B.P. (2007). What's killing American honey bees? PLoS Biol *5*, e168.

Olefsky, J.M., and Glass, C.K. (2010). Macrophages, inflammation, and insulin resistance. Annu. Rev. Physiol. *72*, 219–246.

Ouchi, N., Parker, J.L., Lugus, J.J., and Walsh, K. (2011). Adipokines in inflammation and metabolic disease. Nat. Rev. Immunol. *11*, 85–97.

Packard, C.J. (2003). Triacylglycerol-rich lipoproteins and the generation of small, dense low-density lipoproteins. Biochem. Soc. Trans. *31*, 1066–1069.

Page, K.A., Chan, O., Arora, J., Belfort-DeAguiar, R., Dzuira, J., Roehmholdt, B., Cline, G.W., Naik, S., Sinha, R., Constable, R.T., et al. (2013). Effects of fructose vs glucose on regional cerebral blood flow in brain regions involved with appetite and reward pathways. JAMA *309*, 63–70.

Palaniappan, U., Starkey, L.J., O'Loughlin, J., and Gray-Donald, K. (2001). Fruit and vegetable consumption is lower and saturated fat intake is higher among Canadians reporting smoking. J. Nutr. *131*, 1952–1958.

Parsons, L.H., and Hurd, Y.L. (2015). Endocannabinoid signalling in reward and addiction. Nat. Rev. Neurosci. *16*, 579–594.

Pawlak, D.B., Kushner, J.A., and Ludwig, D.S. (2004). Effects of dietary glycaemic index on adiposity, glucose homoeostasis, and plasma lipids in animals. Lancet Lond. Engl. *364*, 778–785.

Peake, J.M., Suzuki, K., Hordern, M., Wilson, G., Nosaka, K., and Coombes, J.S. (2005). Plasma cytokine changes in relation to exercise intensity and muscle damage. Eur. J. Appl. Physiol. *95*, 514–521.

Pedersen, B.K., and Febbraio, M.A. (2012). Muscles, exercise and obesity: skeletal muscle as a secretory organ. Nat. Rev. Endocrinol. *8*, 457–465.

Piazza, P.V., Rougé-Pont, F., Deroche, V., Maccari, S., Simon, H., and Moal, M.L. (1996). Glucocorticoids have state-dependent stimulant effects on the mesencephalic dopaminergic transmission. Proc. Natl. Acad. Sci. *93*, 8716–8720.

Power, M.L., and Schulkin, J. (2008). Anticipatory physiological regulation in feeding biology: cephalic phase responses. Appetite *50*, 194–206.

Power, M.L., and Schulkin, J. (2013). The evolution of obesity (Baltimore: JHU Press).

Powley, T.L., and Phillips, R.J. (2004). Gastric satiation is volumetric, intestinal satiation is nutritive. Physiol. Behav. *82*, 69–74.

Rada, P., Avena, N.M., and Hoebel, B.G. (2005). Daily bingeing on sugar repeatedly releases dopamine in the accumbens shell. Neuroscience *134*, 737–744.

Ravussin, E., and Bogardus, C. (1989). Relationship of genetics, age, and physical fitness to daily energy expenditure and fuel utilization. Am. J. Clin. Nutr. *49*, 968–975.

Rebello, S.A., and van Dam, R.M. (2013). Coffee consumption and cardiovascular health: getting to the heart of the matter. Curr. Cardiol. Rep. *15*, 403.

Rizos, E.C., Ntzani, E.E., Bika, E., Kostapanos, M.S., and Elisaf, M.S. (2012). Association between omega-3 fatty acid supplementation and risk of major cardiovascular disease events: a systematic review and meta-analysis. JAMA *308*, 1024–1033.

Robinson, M.J.F., and Berridge, K.C. (2013). Instant transformation of learned repulsion into motivational "wanting." Curr. Biol. *23*, 282–289.

Rocha, V.Z., and Libby, P. (2009). Obesity, inflammation, and atherosclerosis. Nat. Rev. Cardiol. *6*, 399–409.

Ropelle, E.R., Flores, M.B., Cintra, D.E., Rocha, G.Z., Pauli, J.R., Morari, J., de Souza, C.T., Moraes, J.C., Prada, P.O., Guadagnini, D., et al. (2010). IL-6 and IL-10 anti-inflammatory activity links exercise to hypothalamic insulin and leptin sensitivity through IKKβ and ER stress inhibition. PLoS Biol. *8*, e1000465.

Rosenbaum, M., and Leibel, R.L. (2010). Adaptive thermogenesis in humans. Int. J. Obes. *34*, S47–S55.

Rosenwasser, A.M., and Turek, F.W. (2015). Neurobiology of circadian rhythm regulation. Sleep Med. Clin. *10*, 403–412.

Ryan, K.K., Woods, S.C., and Seeley, R.J. (2012). Central nervous system mechanisms linking the consumption of palatable high-fat diets to the defense of greater adiposity. Cell Metab. *15*, 137–149.

Samraj, A.N., Pearce, O.M.T., Läubli, H., Crittenden, A.N., Bergfeld, A.K., Banda, K., Gregg, C.J., Bingman, A.E., Secrest, P., Diaz, S.L., et al. (2015). A red meat-derived glycan promotes inflammation and cancer progression. Proc. Natl. Acad. Sci. *112*, 542–547.

Sanborn, M., Kerr, K.J., Sanin, L.H., Cole, D.C., Bassil, K.L., and Vakil, C. (2007). Non-cancer health effects of pesticides: systematic review and implications for family doctors. Can. Fam. Physician *53*, 1712–1720.

Scheer, F.A., Hilton, M.F., Mantzoros, C.S., and Shea, S.A. (2009). Adverse metabolic and cardio-vascular consequences of circadian misalignment. Proc. Natl. Acad. Sci. *106*, 4453–4458.

Schleifer, D. (2012). The perfect solution: how trans fats became the healthy replacement for satu-rated fats. Technol. Cult. *53*, 94–119.

Schoeller, D.A., Cella, L.K., Sinha, M.K., and Caro, J.F. (1997). Entrainment of the diurnal rhythm of plasma leptin to meal timing. J. Clin. Invest. *100*, 1882–1887.

Schoenfeld, J.D., and Ioannidis, J.P. (2013). Is everything we eat associated with cancer? A system-atic cookbook review. Am. J. Clin. Nutr. *97*, 127–134.

Schwabe, L., Tegenthoff, M., Höffken, O., and Wolf, O.T. (2010). Concurrent glucocorticoid and noradrenergic activity shifts instrumental behavior from goal-directed to habitual control. J. Neurosci. *30*, 8190–8196.

Sellmann, C., Priebs, J., Landmann, M., Degen, C., Engstler, A.J., Jin, C.J., Gärttner, S., Spruss, A., Huber, O., and Bergheim, I. (2015). Diets rich in fructose, fat or fructose and fat alter intesti-nal barrier function and lead to the development of nonalcoholic fatty liver disease over time. J. Nutr. Biochem. *26*, 1183–1192.

Sender, R., Fuchs, S., and Milo, R. (2016). Are we really vastly outnumbered? Revisiting the ratio of bacterial to host cells in humans. Cell *164*, 337–340.

Seok, J., Warren, H.S., Cuenca, A.G., Mindrinos, M.N., Baker, H.V., Xu, W., Richards, D.R., McDonald-Smith, G.P., Gao, H., Hennessy, L., et al. (2013). Genomic responses in mouse models poorly mimic human inflammatory diseases. Proc. Natl. Acad. Sci. *110*, 3507–3512.

Seufert, V., Ramankutty, N., and Foley, J.A. (2012). Comparing the yields of organic and conven-tional agriculture. Nature *485*, 229–232.

Shenkin, A. (2006a). The key role of micronutrients. Clin. Nutr. Edinb. Scotl. *25*, 1–13.

Shenkin, A. (2006b). Micronutrients in health and disease. Postgrad. Med. J. *82*, 559–567.

Shi, H., Kokoeva, M.V., Inouye, K., Tzameli, I., Yin, H., and Flier, J.S. (2006). TLR4 links innate immunity and fatty acid-induced insulin resistance. J. Clin. Invest. *116*, 3015–3025.

Sinha, M.K., Ohannesian, J.P., Heiman, M.L., Kriauciunas, A., Stephens, T.W., Magosin, S., Marco, C., and Caro, J.F. (1996). Nocturnal rise of leptin in lean, obese, and non-insulin-dependent diabetes mellitus subjects. J. Clin. Invest. *97*, 1344–1347.

Siri-Tarino, P.W., Sun, Q., Hu, F.B., and Krauss, R.M. (2010). Saturated fat, carbohydrate, and car-diovascular disease. Am. J. Clin. Nutr. *91*, 502–509.

Slavin, J. (2013). Fiber and prebiotics: mechanisms and health benefits. Nutrients *5*, 1417–1435.

Smith, P.M., Howitt, M.R., Panikov, N., Michaud, M., Gallini, C.A., Bohlooly-Y, M., Glickman, J.N., and Garrett, W.S. (2013). The microbial metabolites, short-chain fatty acids, regulate colonic Treg cell homeostasis. Science *341*, 569–573.

Smith-Spangler, C., Brandeau, M.L., Hunter, G.E., Bavinger, J.C., Pearson, M., Eschbach, P.J., Sundaram, V., Liu, H., Schirmer, P., Stave, C., et al. (2012). Are organic foods safer or healthier than conventional alternatives? A systematic review. Ann. Intern. Med. *157*, 348–366.

Sniderman, A.D., Scantlebury, T., and Cianflone, K. (2001). Hypertriglyceridemic hyperapoB: the unappreciated atherogenic dyslipoproteinemia in type 2 diabetes mellitus. Ann. Intern. Med. *135*, 447–459.

Sonnenburg, E.D., and Sonnenburg, J.L. (2014). Starving our microbial self: the deleterious consequences of a diet deficient in microbiota-accessible carbohydrates. Cell Metab. *20*, 779–786.

Sonnenburg, J.L., and Bäckhed, F. (2016). Diet–microbiota interactions as moderators of human metabolism. Nature *535*, 56–64.

de Souza, R.J., Mente, A., Maroleanu, A., Cozma, A.I., Ha, V., Kishibe, T., Uleryk, E., Budylowski, P., Schünemann, H., Beyene, J., et al. (2015). Intake of saturated and trans unsaturated fatty acids and risk of all-cause mortality, cardiovascular disease, and type 2 diabetes: systematic review and meta-analysis of observational studies. BMJ *351*, h3978.

Spruss, A., Kanuri, G., Wagnerberger, S., Haub, S., Bischoff, S.C., and Bergheim, I. (2009). Toll-like receptor 4 is involved in the development of fructose-induced hepatic steatosis in mice. Hepatology *50*, 1094–1104.

Spruss, A., Kanuri, G., Stahl, C., Bischoff, S.C., and Bergheim, I. (2012). Metformin protects against the development of fructose-induced steatosis in mice: role of the intestinal barrier function. Lab. Invest. *92*, 1020–1032.

Starkie, R. (2003). Exercise and IL-6 infusion inhibit endotoxin-induced TNF-alpha production in humans. FASEB J. *17*, 884–6.

Stefka, A.T., Feehley, T., Tripathi, P., Qiu, J., McCoy, K., Mazmanian, S.K., Tjota, M.Y., Seo, G.-Y., Cao, S., Theriault, B.R., et al. (2014). Commensal bacteria protect against food allergen sensitization. Proc. Natl. Acad. Sci. *111*, 13145–13150.

Stenvers, D.J., Jonkers, C.F., Fliers, E., Bisschop, P.H.L.T., and Kalsbeek, A. (2012). Nutrition and the circadian timing system. In Kalsbeek, A., Merrow, M., Roenneberg, T., and Foster, R.G. (eds) Progress in brain research vol. 199 (Amsterdam: Elsevier).

Stephen, A.M., and Cummings, J.H. (1980). The microbial contribution to human faecal mass. J. Med. Microbiol. *13*, 45–56.

Stolarz-Skrzypek, K., Kuznetsova, T., Thijs, L., Tikhonoff, V., Seidlerová, J., Richart, T., Jin, Y., Olszanecka, A., Malyutina, S., Casiglia, E., et al. (2011). Fatal and nonfatal outcomes, incidence of hypertension, and blood pressure changes in relation to urinary sodium excretion. JAMA *305*, 1777–1785.

Stote, K.S., Baer, D.J., Spears, K., Paul, D.R., Harris, G.K., Rumpler, W.V., Strycula, P., Najjar, S.S., Ferrucci, L., Ingram, D.K., et al. (2007). A controlled trial of reduced meal frequency without caloric restriction in healthy, normal-weight, middle-aged adults. Am. J. Clin. Nutr. *85*, 981–988.

Sturm, R., and Hattori, A. (2013). Morbid obesity rates continue to rise rapidly in the United States. Int. J. Obes. 2005 *37*, 889–891.

Suez, J., Korem, T., Zeevi, D., Zilberman-Schapira, G., Thaiss, C.A., Maza, O., Israeli, D., Zmora, N., Gilad, S., Weinberger, A., et al. (2014). Artificial sweeteners induce glucose intolerance by altering the gut microbiota. Nature *514*, 181–6.

Sun, Q. (2012). Red meat consumption and mortality: results from 2 prospective cohort studies. Arch. Intern. Med. *172*, 555.

Suter, P.M., and Tremblay, A. (2005). Is alcohol consumption a risk factor for weight gain and obesity? Crit. Rev. Clin. Lab. Sci. *42*, 197–227.

Takao, K., and Miyakawa, T. (2015). Genomic responses in mouse models greatly mimic human inflammatory diseases. Proc. Natl. Acad. Sci. U. S. A. *112*, 1167–1172.

Tang, W.H.W., Wang, Z., Levison, B.S., Koeth, R.A., Britt, E.B., Fu, X., Wu, Y., and Hazen, S.L. (2013). Intestinal microbial metabolism of phosphatidylcholine and cardiovascular risk. N. Engl. J. Med. *368*, 1575–1584.

Taubes, G. (2010). Why we get fat: and what to do about it (New York: Anchor).

Tchernof, A., and Després, J.-P. (2013). Pathophysiology of human visceral obesity: an update. Physiol. Rev. *93*, 359–404.

Teff, K.L., Elliott, S.S., Tschöp, M., Kieffer, T.J., Rader, D., Heiman, M., Townsend, R.R., Keim, N.L., D'Alessio, D., and Havel, P.J. (2004). Dietary fructose reduces circulating insulin and leptin, attenuates postprandial suppression of ghrelin, and increases triglycerides in women. J. Clin. Endocrinol. Metab. *89*, 2963–2972.

Thaiss, C.A., Zeevi, D., Levy, M., Segal, E., and Elinav, E. (2015). A day in the life of the metaorganism: diurnal rhythms of the intestinal microbiome and its host. Gut Microbes *6*, 137–142.

Thaiss, C.A., Zmora, N., Levy, M., and Elinav, E. (2016). The microbiome and innate immunity. Nature *535*, 65–74.

Tournier, A., and Louis-Sylvestre, J. (1991). Effect of the physical state of a food on subsequent intake in human subjects. Appetite *16*, 17–24.

Touyz, R.M. (2004). Reactive oxygen species, vascular oxidative stress, and redox signaling in hypertension: what is the clinical significance? Hypertension *44*, 248–252.

Tremaroli, V., and Bäckhed, F. (2012). Functional interactions between the gut microbiota and host metabolism. Nature *489*, 242–249.

Troisi, R.J., Heinold, J.W., Vokonas, P.S., and Weiss, S.T. (1991). Cigarette smoking, dietary intake, and physical activity: effects on body fat distribution -- the Normative Aging Study. Am. J. Clin. Nutr. *53*, 1104–1111.

Trompette, A., Gollwitzer, E.S., Yadava, K., Sichelstiel, A.K., Sprenger, N., Ngom-Bru, C., Blanchard, C., Junt, T., Nicod, L.P., Harris, N.L., et al. (2014). Gut microbiota metabolism of dietary fiber influences allergic airway disease and hematopoiesis. Nat. Med. *20*, 159–166.

Tuomilehto, J., Jousilahti, P., Rastenyte, D., Moltchanov, V., Tanskanen, A., Pietinen, P., and Nissinen, A. (2001). Urinary sodium excretion and cardiovascular mortality in Finland: a prospective study. The Lancet *357*, 848–851.

Turnbaugh, P.J., Ley, R.E., Mahowald, M.A., Magrini, V., Mardis, E.R., and Gordon, J.I. (2006). An obesity-associated gut microbiome with increased capacity for energy harvest. Nature *444*, 1027–1131.

Ulluwishewa, D., Anderson, R.C., McNabb, W.C., Moughan, P.J., Wells, J.M., and Roy, N.C. (2011). Regulation of tight junction permeability by intestinal bacteria and dietary components. J. Nutr. *141*, 769–776.

Urban, L.E., Dallal, G.E., Robinson, L.M., Ausman, L.M., Saltzman, E., and Roberts, S.B. (2010). The accuracy of stated energy contents of reduced-energy, commercially prepared foods. J. Am. Diet. Assoc. *110*, 116–123.

Urban, L.E., McCrory, M.A., Dallal, G.E., Das, S.K., Saltzman, E., Weber, J.L., and Roberts, S.B. (2011). Accuracy of stated energy contents of restaurant foods. JAMA *306*, 287–293.

Urgert, R., and Katan, M.B. (1997). The cholesterol-raising factor from coffee beans. Annu. Rev. Nutr. *17*, 305–324.

Vijay-Kumar, M., Aitken, J.D., Carvalho, F.A., Cullender, T.C., Mwangi, S., Srinivasan, S., Sitaraman, S.V., Knight, R., Ley, R.E., and Gewirtz, A.T. (2010). Metabolic syndrome and altered gut microbiota in mice lacking Toll-like receptor 5. Science *328*, 228–231.

Vrieze, A., Van Nood, E., Holleman, F., Salojärvi, J., Kootte, R.S., Bartelsman, J.F.W.M., Dallinga–Thie, G.M., Ackermans, M.T., Serlie, M.J., Oozeer, R., et al. (2012). Transfer of intestinal microbiota from lean donors increases insulin sensitivity in individuals with metabolic syndrome. Gastroenterology *143*, 913–916.e7.

Walker, R.W., Dumke, K.A., and Goran, M.I. (2014). Fructose content in popular beverages made with and without high-fructose corn syrup. Nutrition *30*, 928–935.

Walsh, C.O., Ebbeling, C.B., Swain, J.F., Markowitz, R.L., Feldman, H.A., and Ludwig, D.S. (2013). Effects of diet composition on postprandial energy availability during weight loss maintenance. PLoS ONE *8*, e58172.

Wang, G.J., Volkow, N.D., Logan, J., Pappas, N.R., Wong, C.T., Zhu, W., Netusil, N., and Fowler, J.S. (2001). Brain dopamine and obesity. Lancet Lond. Engl. *357*, 354–357.

Wang, Z., Klipfell, E., Bennett, B.J., Koeth, R., Levison, B.S., DuGar, B., Feldstein, A.E., Britt, E.B., Fu, X., Chung, Y.-M., et al. (2011). Gut flora metabolism of phosphatidylcholine promotes cardiovascular disease. Nature *472*, 57–63.

Wansink, B. (2004). Environmental factors that increase the food intake and consumption volume of unknowing consumers. Annu. Rev. Nutr. *24*, 455–479.

Wansink, B. (2014). Slim by design: mindless eating solutions for everyday life (New York, NY: William Morrow & Company).

Wansink, B., and Chandon, P. (2014). Slim by design: redirecting the accidental drivers of mindless overeating. J. Consum. Psychol. *24*, 413–431.

Wansink, B., Painter, J.E., and Lee, Y.-K. (2006). The office candy dish: proximity's influence on estimated and actual consumption. Int. J. Obes. *30*, 871–875.

Wen, L., Ley, R.E., Volchkov, P.Y., Stranges, P.B., Avanesyan, L., Stonebraker, A.C., Hu, C., Wong, F.S., Szot, G.L., Bluestone, J.A., et al. (2008). Innate immunity and intestinal microbiota in the development of Type 1 diabetes. Nature *455*, 1109–1113.

Whitman, W.B., Coleman, D.C., and Wiebe, W.J. (1998). Prokaryotes: the unseen majority. Proc. Natl. Acad. Sci. *95*, 6578–6583.

Willis, L.H., Slentz, C.A., Bateman, L.A., Shields, A.T., Piner, L.W., Bales, C.W., Houmard, J.A., and Kraus, W.E. (2012). Effects of aerobic and/or resistance training on body mass and fat mass in overweight or obese adults. J. Appl. Physiol. Bethesda Md 1985 *113*, 1831–1837.

Wing, R.R., and Jeffery, R.W. (2001). Food provision as a strategy to promote weight loss. Obes. Res. *9*, 271S–275S.

Winkler, J.T. (2005). The fundamental flaw in obesity research. Obes. Rev. *6*, 199–202.

Wise, R.A. (2004). Dopamine, learning and motivation. Nat. Rev. Neurosci. *5*, 483–494.

Wren, A.M., and Bloom, S.R. (2007). Gut hormones and appetite control. Gastroenterology *132*, 2116–2130.

Yang, X., and Ruan, H.-B. (2015). Neuronal control of adaptive thermogenesis. Front. Endocrinol. *6*, 149.

Yore, M.M., Syed, I., Moraes-Vieira, P.M., Zhang, T., Herman, M.A., Homan, E.A., Patel, R.T., Lee, J., Chen, S., Peroni, O.D., et al. (2014). Discovery of a class of endogenous mammalian lipids with anti-diabetic and anti-inflammatory effects. Cell *159*, 318–332.

Zeevi, D., Korem, T., Zmora, N., Israeli, D., Rothschild, D., Weinberger, A., Ben-Yacov, O., Lador, D., Avnit-Sagi, T., Lotan-Pompan, M., et al. (2015). Personalized nutrition by prediction of glycemic responses. Cell *163*, 1079–1094.

Zeisel, S.H., Mar, M.-H., Howe, J.C., and Holden, J.M. (2003). Concentrations of choline-containing compounds and betaine in common foods. J. Nutr. *133*, 1302–1307.

Zhang, X., Zhang, G., Zhang, H., Karin, M., Bai, H., and Cai, D. (2008). Hypothalamic IKKβ/NF-κB and ER stress link overnutrition to energy imbalance and obesity. Cell *135*, 61–73.

Index

Lightning Source UK Ltd.
Milton Keynes UK
UKHW021432061118
331870UK00003B/402/P